“If you want true healthcare solutio[illegible] ties, you’ll find them in ***The Cure***. Seth Denson provides a beacon of hope for an industry drowning in a sea of noise. Straightforward and results-driven, the message in ***The Cure*** provides the path we need to fix the U.S. healthcare and health insurance systems.”

—Andy Neary, Healthcare Strategist, Business Coach, Speaker, Author

“Seth Denson is my go-to guest on health care issues. Just as he does on my radio show, in ***The Cure***, he explains the issues that have created problems in our health care system in a way that’s clear to understand AND he details actual solutions.”

—Jeff Angelo, Talk Show Host, Newsradio 1040 WHO

“I strongly recommend ***The Cure: A Blueprint for Solving America’s Healthcare Crisis***. Anyone can relate to *Chapter 6: “The Doctor Can See You Now”*. While the topic can make your blood boil, Seth has logical solutions. While covering various issues and topics in the health industry, I’ve interviewed Seth multiple times throughout the years. His approach to solving healthcare is straightforward and makes a complex issue easy and interesting to understand.”

—Audrey Morton, KTRH News Reporter

“As he has many times as a guest on my show, Seth Denson lays out a clear, concise and sensible way to fix America’s health care mess. ‘Health care for all’ are just words. In this book, Denson offers what the real meaning of that phrase should be. Health care is a ‘hot button’ issue in the 2020 elections. ***The Cure*** is a blueprint to what health care should be for all of us.”

—Ken Broo, Talk Show Host, 700 WLW

“Solid. Paradigm shifting view and insight on the health care market. Wake up Washington, here is your blueprint.”

—Mark Turner, Founder and CEO of N2Success

"Healthcare is a complex issue with significant possible ramifications. In ***The Cure***, Seth outlines specific objectives that will yield positive results for all Americans. He is truly a modern day Lorax for healthcare."

—Jeff Crilly, Emmy Award Winning Reporter

"Seth Denson's book, ***The Cure***, uses clear-headed rationality to show that US Healthcare System improvement requires 1) different government regulation and 2) patient behavior change. I think that is right. ***The Cure*** says improvement will NOT come from health insurers, hospitals, doctors or pharmaceutical companies. I think that is right too. Want to change healthcare? Follow ***The Cure's*** directive."

—Eric Bricker, MD, Chief Medical Officer AHealthcareZ, Former Co-Founder Compass Professional Health Services

THE CURE

A BLUEPRINT FOR SOLVING AMERICA'S HEALTH CARE CRISIS

SETH DENSON

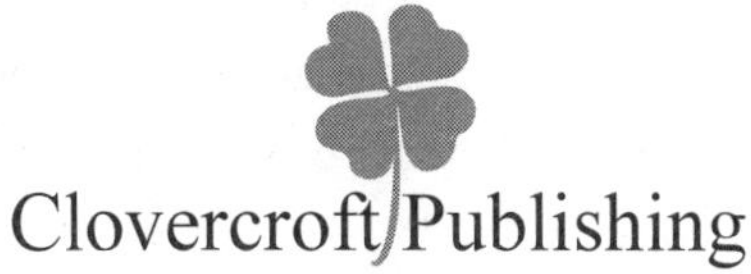

The Cure: A Blueprint for Solving America's Healthcare Crisis

Published by Clovercroft Publishing, Franklin, Tennessee

Edited by Leroy Titus Elliott

Cover Design by Nelly Sanchez

Interior Design by Adept Content Solutions

Printed in the United States of America

978-1-950892-07-5

Contents

This book is dedicated to my mother and father, Elaine and Rick Denson, who instilled within my brothers and me the inherent belief that it was our duty and calling to improve the lives of others. It is my hope that the words found on the pages within this book do just that, and that, through them, lives will be impacted in a positive way.

Acknowledgments

This book is well over 100 pages long. For me to take the time to name and properly thank all those that have influenced me in both my development and the writing of this project would take 100 more. This book has been a labor of love , and it has been influenced by so many people and experiences in order to wrap words around thoughts and ideas. I won't be able to name them all or thank them properly, but there are a few that I must acknowledge.

First and foremost, my beautiful wife, **Jenna**. Without your love, support, and patience, this book would have never come to fruition. You have been a constant support throughout my career and have always encouraged me to follow my passion. You are my rock and my reason. I've loved you since the day we met, and I will love you all the remaining days of my life. Thank you for so much more than I can ever say.

To my beautiful **children**. You have given me a new purpose to see and make the world a better place. You fill my heart with joy and have taught me what love is and what it truly can be.

To my parents, **Rick** and **Elaine**. Everything good about me has been the result of our dedication and commitment to our family.

To my other parents, **Jeff** and **Tracy**. You raised an amazing daughter whom I'm so blessed to call my wife; moreover, you welcomed me with open arms into your family and became not in-laws to me, but rather another mom and dad. For your love and support and encouragement, I will be forever grateful.

To my two grandmothers. First, to my paternal grandmother, Wanda Denson, who taught me the beauty of communication through the written word. And second, to my maternal grandmother, Karen Ivy, who taught me to always strive for knowledge and never stop learning.

To my extended family, my **brothers** and **sisters** (in-law or not). You have always shown your love and have been there for me when I needed an ear to bend. I love you all.

To my business partner, **John Powter**. You took a young energetic no-knowledge entrepreneur under your wing and have made me a better friend, boss, and businessman. I'm forever in your debt.

To my executive team at GDP Advisors, **John** and **Carrie**. You patiently supported me throughout the writing of this book and allowed my attention to veer away from other duties and picked up the slack in my absence. Thank you.

To my entire **staff/team** at GDP. You all inspire me each and every day. You are truly a group of professionals driven to make people's lives better. You certainly make mine better each and every day.

To **Larry Linne**, my mentor, coach, and friend. You have led me down a path of success and instilled in me the desire to be better each and every day. Thank you for your leadership and friendship.

To **Luke Grizzaffi**. You taught me what it means to really care about those who look to us for counsel.

To my "**Midland**" boys. We've shared a lifetime of friendship, and as iron sharpens iron, you have been there for me through good times and bad.

To the team at OnFire Books, **Tammy**, **Tiarra**, **Sharon**, **Nelly**, and so many more. You've shown me how to take my thoughts and ideas and put them into words. Words are currency, and you've taught me how to spend that currency well. Together we will change lives.

And last but certainly not least, to **Andrew Clark**, my right hand and friend. Without your dedication and commitment, this book would have never been completed. Your contribution is found throughout the research, ideas, solutions, and words within these pages, and together we will change the world.

For Emersen, Arabella, and Connor

Unless someone like you cares a whole awful lot,
nothing is going to get better. It's not.

—Dr. Seuss, *The Lorax*

Foreword

There is a classic comedy skit from *Monty Python & the Holy Grail* centered on a group of people suffering from sickness and health problems. In their search for the cause of their woes, they come to the conclusion that there must be witches in their midst. In their efforts to identify who among them is the witch, they determine, through a hilarious dialogue along with some ridiculous comparisons, how they might identify who among them is the witch. The crowd gets more and more worked up, as they encourage each other in their beliefs and convictions. They cheer "Burn the witch," as they realize they have found their culprit (which is ultimately based on nonsense). They believe the problem will now be solved! They found a witch, and they can rid themselves of it. They will no longer be sick!

This scene often comes to mind when I read comments and opinions on social media and the news about health care or when I listen to individuals talk about it. People are so frustrated with the cost and availability of health care that they just want to find an answer, regardless of how nonsensical some of the solutions might be.

It is human nature to eliminate a fear or a problem so we can be safe and feel secure in our lives.

Health care is clearly one of these problems that need to be solved. The costs are continuing to go up, and access to appropriate care seems to be less and less available.

In a country where the doctors are the best in the world, where medicines are the highest quality and have the greatest research behind them, and where resources are the most advanced, we have some of the poorest outcomes, lowest levels of appropriate access, and a steady decline in the overall health of our citizens.

THIS IS A REAL PROBLEM.

However, we keep attacking the problem with political partisanship and ignorance. We are given "solutions" set forward by politicians who are monetarily and politically motivated and who have little to no experience with the health care industry. Yet we will listen to a sound bite and make their idea our health care solution mantra! Most people come to conclusions that they don't truly even understand. They get the surface message and latch onto it with conviction and don't understand the complete cause and effect of that answer. Thus, we yell, "Burn the witch!"

It is time for us to understand the problem(s) of health care in America with depth, sound logic, nonpartisanship, no sound bites, and with mindfulness.

The Cure is exactly that—a cure for what truly ails us in health care in the United States. It is the cure for solving health care. It is complex. It addresses deep cause and effect. It gives answers that are hard to accomplish but that are "right."

Seth Denson has given us the answers that will require all three stakeholders (consumers, health care providers, government) to understand the problems in health care and to join together to solve them.

I have watched Seth over the years as he has taken on this challenge of understanding the problem and the potential solutions. He has been thoughtful and nonpartisan, and he has dug deep into cause and effect. He has thought through the logic beyond the social media and the political crowd. Seth has the passion to solve this problem and the intellect to bring truth to the mob.

I believe that if this book was read by everyone in America, we would quickly solve the problems at the core in a thoughtful manner and with logic that is mindful and real.

Let's increase our perceived intelligence and lose the arguments of ignorance that are driven by sound bites. You can make a difference if you read and understand what Seth offers in this book, and then act on it!

I encourage you to read on ...

Larry Linne
CEO InCite Performance Group
Chairman of Intellectual Innovations
Author of *Brand Aid*
Author of *Make the Noise Go Away*

A Note from the Author

Dear Reader,

I firmly believe that the future of health care is up to all of us, and I hope that, by the end of this book, you will, too. There is a saying, "*Be the change*," by Gandhi, and, in the case of healthcare, it's true. Each one of us has a great responsibility to take back control of our health care and be *The Cure*. I love the story of Dr. Seuss's *The Lorax* where a single character is doing all he can to save the powerless from the destruction and devastation caused by unbridled greed and power. In the end, the Lorax succeeds because of the actions of one. American scientist Margaret Mead once said, "*Never doubt that a small group of thoughtful, committed citizens can change the world; indeed, it's the only thing that ever has.*" It is my hope that the ideas shared within the pages of this book can ignite a movement. But even if only a few take up the call, it might be enough to change the world. Thank you for reading.

—Seth Denson

CHAPTER 1

In Need of Treatment

Health care is a drug. In a world of addictions, including caffeine, tobacco, opioids, and social media, we are a society influenced by our modern dependencies. The challenge with many vices is we often don't even realize when we are hooked. It wasn't always this way, and dependencies are not always addictions. I depend on water and air in the same way that, to live life to the fullest, I depend on health care. However, over the past century, the United States has perverted the way health care is delivered, accessed, financed, and consumed. As such, the health care industry, acting the role of a drug dealer, has made addicts of us all.

Chances are you've experienced challenges while navigating the health care system, or you know someone who has. How have unexpected bills and confusion about what your insurance does and doesn't cover impacted your life? How about insurance networks? Do you really know how to determine what's in and out of network? Should the government come in and simply take the entire thing over? Is that the only way out? Health care is at the forefront of many minds and has been an issue of continual debate in our homes, in the workplace, and throughout our politics.

The purpose of this book is to discuss where American health care is right now, how we got here, and where we are heading. The situation is dire, to be sure, but don't let that discourage you; we can alter our course and navigate a different outcome. We can break the addiction and reestablish a health care system meant to positively impact the lives of our citizens, without destroying businesses or establishing oppressive price fixing.

I've been part of the health care industry for nearly twenty years, working in various facets, and believe me: I've seen it all. I've seen the good sides of health care, things like the delivery of new life or times when patients endure hard times and emerge stronger and healthier on the other end. I've witnessed surgery and later physical therapy that led to a wonderful outcome and a better quality of life. I've seen the ugly, too—when people go through the pain of losing a loved one or unnecessary testing and treatments. I've known those who have gone bankrupt while caring for their loved ones, while hospitals concern themselves more with money than care and procedures and prescriptions are handed out for no reason other than to raise the bottom line.

And it's because of the ugliness that we must find a cure, all the while preserving what is good and great about our system. It's time for an intervention: a serious conversation to break us from the negative aspects of the health care system and instead "reformat" a system that achieves great things, serves the masses, and sustains our pursuit of happiness. But how? This isn't some friend who lost their path; this is the American Medical Complex, an industry so large it makes up a sixth of the US economy, impacts millions of jobs, and has the single largest lobbying group in Washington. Where do we even start with a system so vast and so vital that to fail could crash the entire American economic engine?

Pundits will tell you that there are many layers to these problems and that those layers are very complex. Some will say it's all about ingenuity, but the United States is responsible for nearly 70 percent of all technological medical advancements throughout the world, yet, according to the World Health Organization, the United States ranks thirty-seventh in overall health, while ranking number one in overall cost (nearly double that of most other First World countries). Infant mortality is nearly double of that in other comparable nations, while the United States ranks nineteenth overall in obesity (with 33.7 percent of the population listed as obese). In addition, with all of the brilliance behind our system, we lose more of our citizens to heart disease, diabetes, and cancer, than we do to all other causes of death combined. Some will say we have an access problem, but we don't. It's not that the single mother with two kids in just about any metro area of the United States can't walk to a street corner to access the health care system, it's that she can't afford it once she's gotten there. So if ingenuity and access aren't the problem, what is it? *Cost*—or dare I say, *profit*. Plain and simple, it's all about the dollar, and while that, in and of itself, can be a challenge, it's not necessarily always a bad thing! I'm a free market capitalist and firmly believe that our economic system in the United States is the greatest on the face of the earth. It is the nature of our system that encourages the advancements and innovations in medicine, but when an I.V. bag costs less than $1 to make but is billed, on average, $546 per unit by hospitals (a 54,000 percent markup), we have a serious problem. Yes, when it comes to one person's health blended with another's profit margin, we can often find ourselves in a conflict of capitalism versus care.

There are numerous books outlining where the system went wrong, and while we will touch on some of those things, the title of this book is *The Cure*, so rest assured that, instead of finger-pointing, we're going to outline ways to actually solve these problems. And, in so doing, we'll address the four influencers of the health care system (the government, the delivery system, the finance/insurance market, and the consumer) and their roles in curing the system as it sits today.

This book does not intend to take a political side or to promote any particular agenda. I've spoken on media outlets endearing themselves to a particular side of the political spectrum—FOX News, NBC, CBS, ABC, and others—and I frequently discuss health care on radio stations big and small: AM, FM, and XM. Inevitably, I have been called out by members of both political parties as advocating the other party's policies (which I tend to find amusing). My hope is that, by the end of this book, you won't know which political affiliation I keep or how I might vote from one election to the next. I say this because the problems within the US health care system are not partisan problems. Diseases don't have a party affiliation, nor should solutions to cure them.

In the same way, this book does not contain a magical, one-step switch to either a single-payer or free-health care-for-all platform; nor does it advocate for a continuance of the system we have now, with crony capitalism run amuck. Those are the cries of the politician, who is trying to secure votes. I'm going to simply "tell it like it is." Here's the truth: we worked hard to build this country, and we will also need to work hard to repair the health care industry. This book is about the small steps that we can take to alter some of the core tenants of the health care system. We will need to reform how care is delivered, how it is financed, how it is advanced, and finally, how it is obtained. Like pieces within a puzzle, we must look at all parts of the health care system to begin to provide solutions to cure it.

CHAPTER 2

Health Care—It's Personal

When I began writing this book, I was told by many that my efforts would be futile, at best. Health care is too big and too complex a problem to solve in one book. While the better part of me might agree with this perspective, I was raised to consider that those crazy enough to think they can change the world are oftentimes the very ones who do. In the same manner, I was also taught that to solve big problems, one must identify the various aspects of that problem, quantify them, and create a plan of action to solve them. Much like when building a house, it must be done brick by brick, with the foundation being your purpose or your "WHY." There must be a blueprint of action to guarantee success at each juncture. I have been in the vocational health care sector most of my adult life—it is "WHAT" I do, but "WHY" I do it has become the internal alarm clock that gets me up in the morning, pushes me to continue to learn, and is the motivation behind writing this book. To better understand my "WHY," and thus my key inspiration behind this project, I'd like to tell you my story and personal interaction with health care.

While I was growing up, our family didn't have health insurance. My father was the pastor of a small church in Midland, Texas, and the congregation operated on a limited budget. For this reason, health insurance for its staff was not an option. By the age of twelve, I would require more than ten surgeries because of a nonlife-threatening medical condition. While minor in nature, these procedures created a significant financial burden on our family. Not realizing the reasoning at the time, I watched as my father would take jobs outside of his role at our church to be able to either obtain health insurance or earn enough money to pay cash for the treatments of my condition. This was the 1980s and the early 1990s, so the ability to access the market without insurance and to negotiate a cash deal was still a viable option—a feat that would be all but impossible in today's health care climate.

Both of my parents were selfless, always putting their family first, others second, and themselves last. While I was growing up, we were not poor, but we didn't have a lot of money, either. I don't recall ever going without; as a matter of fact, I always thought we must have had significant means, given that my brothers and I always seemed to have more than we needed or really wanted. We were rich—not in the monetary sense but rather in that we had two parents who loved each other, who loved us, and who shared their love with us.

Contrary to the belief of those that know me best, I did not grow up with aspirations of being in the health insurance finance and health care industry. While other kids were wearing superman capes, fire fighter helmets, or police badges, I wasn't wearing a suit and carrying a briefcase ... okay, maybe I was, but not with the idea that it would lead me to the career I have now. Like most children,

I dreamed of being a policeman, a cowboy like John Wayne, or a fighter jet pilot (it was the 1980s, and *Top Gun* was a big deal). Yes, my childhood visions of the adult version of me were similar in nature to those of most kids, I suppose; however, there was always something within me that liked to fix things.

My mother loves telling the story of the time when I was three years old. I would go outside, get in my little red foot-powered car, with my toy tool bag, and proceed to go door to door down the block on the street on which I grew up. My purpose for this adventure was to visit our neighbors, asking if they had anything that needed "fixin'" (as we say in Texas). Obviously, at three years old, my capacity limited my ability to actually accomplish any task associated with home improvement, but our neighbors were gracious enough to let me try—and usually to let me think I'd provided them with high-quality service. Regardless, the idea of repairing that which was broken has always been part of my core.

By college, I was, I suppose, like many adolescents, attempting to find my purpose and place in the world. It was actually my college counselor who helped guide me into the health insurance space by encouraging me to pursue something I enjoyed. It's not that I enjoyed insurance (who does); rather, I enjoyed playing golf, and, per her recommendation, I began asking those who got to play a lot of golf what they did for a living. I would focus my inquiries towards those who not only got to play what I would consider to be an acceptable amount of golf but also, specifically, those who got do so throughout the week—during working hours. An overwhelming number of those with whom I engaged informed me they were in the insurance business. With this helpful information in hand, insurance became the "WHAT" that would allow me to pursue my "WHY"—golf. Numerous jobs, rounds of golf, and more than a decade would pass before my "WHY" would become what it is today.

By the time I was thirty, I had worked numerous jobs throughout the health insurance market, my first as a junior associate with small agency in Midland, Texas, where I grew up. I would leave that job a year later to start my own firm, and, after a few long years with very little success, I took a position with a national Fortune 500 insurance carrier. It was this job where I learned about underwriting, rating methodologies, insurance profit margins, marketing strategies, and the many tentacles and motivations within the health care system. The knowledge I gained at the national carrier provided me with the opportunity to join a consulting firm where, at twenty-nine, I would find myself about to be named a partner. I had, so I thought, found my place in this world and was even able to find time for a round or two of golf each week.

It was a Thursday—I'll never forget—when all my "plans" changed. December 30, 2010, was a day that would end one season and begin a new one, but one more focused and determined than ever. On the eve of being named partner at the firm that I had called home for nearly five years, I was informed by the existing partners that they had, instead, decided to sell the organization to a national brokerage. Looking back, I don't fault them for their decision—the employee benefits and health insurance landscape was (and still is) in a season of massive uncertainty. Our firm was small but successful, and out of a desire to maintain that success, the leaders of our firm believed the best option was to align ourselves with a larger, more powerful, and more influential organization. I myself was crushed. Sitting in the conference room as I learned the news of the coming acquisition, I could not fight my emotions. It was as if a family was breaking apart and with it, all my plans for the future. I had grown to love our organization, the people within it, and what we stood for. Times were changing, however, and I was not prepared for this change.

Given the speed by which the acquisition was to take place, I did not have time to plan for alternatives. Twelve short hours after I learned of our firm's coming change, the announcement was made and went into effect two short days later. While I was deciding whether or not to join the larger firm that was acquiring us or to determine my alternative next steps, something was mentioned that dramatically changed my career course and life goals. During the brief window of time that I had to make a career decision about my future, it was said to me that if I were to join the larger, more powerful firm, I would "make more money that I ever dreamed possible."

It was at that moment that I flashed back to a conversation that my father and I had almost twelve years prior. It happened in the center field of a baseball stadium in Abilene, Texas, during my senior year of high school. I was preparing to play what would be the last baseball game of my life, and as was part of the pregame routine, my father and I would visit while I stretched and got prepared for the game. Much like the career situation in which I found myself in 2010, twelve years earlier, I was also struggling to make an impacting decision in my life, but this time, it was the decision about which college to attend and whether or not to continue my baseball career. While on that field in West Texas, my father said something to me that I had forgotten, until that fateful December afternoon in 2010. He said, "Whatever decisions you make, promise me this—never chase money, because you'll find that you will never catch it."

Up to that point in my career, I was focused on the title, a country club membership, and the dollar. How high I could climb the ladder, what status I could obtain, and how much money I could make. I don't believe I was arrogant or pretentious, but my purpose lacked proper focus. My "WHAT" was obvious, but my "WHY" required some adjusting.

I appreciated the statement "more money than I ever dreamed possible" that was made to me as I struggled with the decision about my next steps. It was those exact words that hurtled me back to the wisdom my father had shared with me regarding money. I had known for some time that our health care system was fractured, but I recognized, in that moment (as if a light switch had been turned on), that I was part of the problem. The health care system was (and still is) benefiting the bottom line of hospitals and providers, insurance companies, and me, the insurance broker, who was compensated for my efforts to stay "in the box" and maintain the status quo. I began thinking differently about the health care system: instead of it being a vehicle to provide me with wealth, I started thinking about those that were truly impacted by it. There were many winners in the current system, but those that the system was meant to serve were often losing. I could change that—I *would* change that. With the unwavering support of my wife, I decided that I would refocus my goals and change my "WHY." I desired to return to the dream I had when I was three years old and to begin the process of "fixin'" things. With a new and fresh purpose and focus, I set out to change the world—but little did I know that I soon would find myself on the receiving end of the health care system, which would take my "WHY" to a whole new level.

For the next year or so, the "struggle" was real. Leaving the firm I'd called home without a real plan of action proved to be challenging. A little more than a year later, I merged my firm with another, and, throughout that merger, I found a business partner (whom I still have today) that also was restructuring his "WHAT" and "WHY." John, my new business partner, added outstanding business leadership experience, which I was lacking, and I brought passion, energy, and vision. We were still searching for our "WHY," but we were determined and motivated.

In 2014, after years of trying, my wife and I welcomed our first child, Emersen, then another, Arabella, in 2015. At eight weeks old, our youngest daughter contracted an illness that threatened her life. We spent the next week at the local children's hospital near where we lived in North Texas, with Arabella in and out of the intensive care unit. There's no greater fear for parents than that of the thought of losing their child. I remember walking the halls of the hospital and seeing families who, unfortunately, found themselves more regularly there than in their actual homes. I recall their sick children and speaking with other fathers, burdened not only about their children but also about the financial impact these illnesses would have on their entire families and whether the funds might run out before their children overcame their condition. It was this real-life, firsthand experience that led me from one who talked about our flawed system to one experiencing it. While Arabella would ultimately recover (and I will be forever grateful to the amazing doctors and nurses who cared for my little girl), in the end, while we were blessed to take our daughter home, we also took with us bills to the tune of more than $100,000. This challenging experience put our easy-to-manage family (and budget) into a tailspin, but while the experience was challenging, because of the ultimate outcome, there's rarely been a happier time in my entire life. I thought often about the financial struggles my parents had as a result of my medical conditions and realized that they likely would not have been able to do what they did in today's health care world (just a few decades later). I knew then that the trajectory of our system had to change. This experience took my "WHY" to a whole new level, and, because of this, my "WHAT" was changing, too.

CHAPTER 3

Where the Solutions Lie

There's an old saying that, in medicine, general practitioners will tell you what ailment you have and specialists will tell you that you have what they treat. There's profit in the problems. The challenge with finding solutions to today's health care system is that often those who are giving recommendations are also those who stand to benefit from their own propositions. It's hard to trust the glass seller when he's the one who put a brick through your window.

In the spring of 2017, while on a return flight home from a business meeting in California, I had the pleasure of sitting next to Dr. Henry "Hank" Foster. To some, the name "Henry Foster" may not sound familiar, but I assure you that, to many, the name means quite a lot. On top of being a renowned OB-GYN and the only black graduate from his class at the University of Arkansas Medical School in 1958, Mr. Foster served as a policy advisor for the Clinton Administration and was President Bill Clinton's nominee to be surgeon general in 1995.

To me, "Hank," as he asked to be called, was my neighbor on a three-hour flight who quickly became a friend. I always look forward to the randomness of potential acquaintances to be met by happenstance on a flight. Sometimes the randomness can prove to be an annoyance, but, in this case, it proved to be an absolute pleasure.

Throughout the course of our brief, although in-depth, conversation, the topic of health care and its current state in the United States came up. When discussing not only legislation like the Affordable Care Act but also the GOP-led congressional attempt at health care reform (which ultimately failed), the American Health Care Act of 2017, Hank said something to me that I will not soon forget. While he claimed that his statement was an adaptation from something said by Winston Churchill, his comment regarding health care in the United States was this: "Americans will almost always do the right thing—so long as they've tried all the wrong things first."

The Wrong Thing

In 2010, the Affordable Care Act was signed into law by President Barack Obama after being passed by both the House of Representatives and the Senate, with not a single Republican vote. This completely partisan piece of legislation, while intending to do some good and with many admirable parts, was, in effect, dead on arrival. With the country so deeply divided on the topic of health care and with the state of US politics so polarized, the need for leaders to come together and work together to fix the health care problem was, and still is, too far from reach. It's not that the ACA was bad all in all but that the law had limited potential for success, because, as is the case with most things, the original draft needed some improvement and the powers that be, who have the ability to improve it, had no desire to do so.

Fast forward to 2017, and the Republican-led House of Representatives passed the American Healthcare Act—the ACA replacement bill—but, this time, without a single Democratic vote. Rather than fix the original broken legislation, the new leadership chose to attempt to repeal it, or at least a large part of it, by means of budgetary reconciliation and, in turn, to put into place a bill that, much like its predecessor, would have had little chance of accomplishing anything. While the Republican plan ultimately failed, because even Republicans couldn't agree on a solution, if it had passed, it would have made very little impact on the underlying issues within our health care system. Both the ACA and the AHCA would not have been effective because they primarily focused on one piece of the problem, health insurance, rather than the entire puzzle. Sure, health insurance is the method by which most Americans access the health care system, but one (health insurance) is not the other (health care). Allow me to explain.

Health Care versus Health Insurance

Nearly twenty years ago, I entered the insurance industry. While studying for my licensing exam, I learned the basic definition of insurance, which is, in effect, the transfer of risk. While this may be the term and the intent, insurance, more specifically health insurance, has become a risk-finance mechanism rather than a risk transference (we'll discuss more about the health insurance industry in a later chapter).

The first and most obvious problem facing the current state of the health care system in the United States is not the financing mechanism, but the system itself. To keep us in the dark on this, pundits and lobbyists have done a phenomenal job of marketing and spin. Take health care and health insurance, for example. To many Americans, these two terms are synonymous when, in reality, they are very different words and have two very different definitions. Health care is, and should be, associated with describing the actual care received by participants in the health care system—for example, doctor visits, surgery, hospitalization, and even prescription drugs are all aspects of health care. Health insurance is the way in which accessing the health care system is financed.

So often I hear people talk about health care reform, but, in reality, as a country, we seem to want only to focus on health insurance reform. If the focus is only on one part of the problem, then the other parts go untouched and unresolved. As we continue to think through the solution to rising health insurance costs, perhaps we should think through the differences between health care and health insurance and begin using those two terms in an appropriate way.

The Obvious Problem that Everyone Seems to Ignore

I've always been fascinated with innovative business leaders—those that seem to have the pulse of their specific industries and therefore are always on the cutting edge. The Dyson organization has always impressed me—not because it has my family so convinced in its superiority that we have sworn off any other brand of vacuum cleaner in our home—but because of their constant ingenuity. Years ago, I read an interview given by the founder of Dyson, in which he outlined the reason for the organization's success. He stated (and I'm sure I'm paraphrasing) that it "focused on the obvious problems that its competitors ignored." How does this apply to the current state of health care in the United States? I'm sure most of us can agree that there are really two legislative teams in the health care battle and that they are most definitely competitors; however, they would serve themselves well by heeding the words of the Dyson founder, in that they should focus on the obvious problem that everyone else in Washington seems to ignore.

Health insurance companies are, for the most part, publicly traded corporations with fiduciary responsibility to their shareholders and not to their insureds. Don't get me wrong; I consider myself a true-blue capitalist, and I believe that organizations must have the right to be profitable ones; however, there is an absolute conflict and adverse incentive for insurance companies in today's climate. Regardless of one's political affiliation or opinion, access to adequate health care in a country as great as the United States should be attainable for all; however, until the Affordable Care Act, it simply was not.

The obvious problem with the ACA, however, is that it did nothing to impact health care; rather, it focused primarily on the financing mechanism, health insurance. (The same could be said for the AHCA, had it passed.) If we can all agree that insurance companies must collect more in premiums than they pay out in claims, then we should also agree that best way to reduce those premiums would be to reduce the cost of what is financed by them. If we agree on this, then we can see that the glaring issue with the ACA was that it focused primarily on the insurance premiums, not the costs driving up those premiums.

Insurance companies—while bemoaning the ACA and its potential impact on them—have actually fared well because of the law. Under the Affordable Care Act, the primary piece that was meant to "reign in" insurance companies was the MLR (medical loss ratio) requirement. The MLR provision of the law stated that insurance companies had to spend a specific percentage of the premiums they collected on actual claims, thus capping their expenses and profit-margin percentages. The MLR ratio was set to be 80 percent to 85 percent (depending on whether the policy was written for an individual, a small group, or a large group). In other words, the ACA stipulates that insurance companies must spend between 80 percent to 85 percent of all premium dollars on the payment of claims. While this may seem like a good idea, as is the case with most ideas, the devil is in the details. What Congress failed to understand was that these billion-dollar organizations are run by pretty savvy business professionals. And if you are one of these business pros and you are likely driven by your ability to impact your shareholders' stock price and if the government set a percentage of profit margin, would you want that percentage to be based on a lower or a higher premium cost? To use an analogy, it's as if the US government said, "We don't care what you charge for the car; we're only going to regulate the interest rate by which it is financed."

The unintended consequence of the ACA was that insurance companies would no longer be interested in driving the actual cost of health care down, as that would, in turn, reduce the actual dollar amount that they could earn. Instead, they needed the cost of health care to rise so that the 15 percent to 20 percent of premiums that they didn't have to use to pay claims would be a higher number. As a result, since the ACA was signed into law on March 23, 2010, the five largest publicly traded insurance companies have seen an average stock price increase over of 200 percent. When you regulate only the percentage of profit but not the specific dollar amount of profit, that dollar amount will likely increase.

The Right Thing

Einstein said that one should make a problem as simple as possible, but no simpler. That there are twelve chapters in this book detailing the struggles and challenges with the health care system is evidence in and of itself that the struggle is a multifaceted one, with many sides that can all be addressed in different ways. Which is why when someone on the news or on the radio or at political rally says, "All we have to do is X, Y, or Z to fix it!" that person is talking nonsense. He or she may have a piece of the puzzle, but that's not enough to see the entire image. There is no one-size-fits-all solution, and, yes, I know it would be so comforting—such a breath of relief—to be able to look to someone or something for the easy answer and not have to think or do any work for ourselves, but that's not going to be the case here.

So let's make this simple. In the end, the problem we have with the American health care system is the price. In general, we don't have a quality-of-care problem in the United States; we don't have an accessibility issue; we have a dollar sign issue. We have a human need for health services; we're going to get sick or hurt, and we want either ourselves or our loved ones to live long and pain-free lives. Health care is essential to these needs and wants. Health care is a service we must have, and it is being leveraged unfairly against us. As will be stated multiple times throughout this book, this is due, in large part, to the lack of transparency in the system, which results in our inability to affect meaningful change, which results in the cost being set not at what the market will bear but at artificially inflated prices that have bankrupted so many and that have resulted in daily crises for many more.

I do not advocate that health care be given away for free. Doctors work incredibly hard for more than a decade to achieve their mastery, and they have a right to be rewarded for their efforts. In the same way, companies that facilitate care are massive organizations that require millions of man-hours per year of administration, tedium, and coordination. They, too, deserve to make a profit. But I do have a problem with the costs, artificially inflated by over 1,000 percent, of some prescription drugs, procedures, and needed care. There needs to be a balance. There needs to be legislation to course-correct some of these issues, and there needs to be a halt to the opaque nature of cost that is enjoyed by these medical companies.

So let us be like doctors ourselves and rule out what we know will not work to arrive at the best possible diagnosis and treatment. It's actually quite simple—it's a matter of economics.

The "economic principle" states that the true cost of something is equal to the number of units consumed multiplied by its price. Business owners have long since known this principle and have applied it to most everything in their businesses. Pizza restaurant owners, for example, know that if the cost of meat or cheese goes up, they will need to think about repricing the pizza or lowering the quantity of pepperoni used. If fuel costs go up, the same pizza restauranteurs might rethink how they manage their delivery routes or where they send out their drivers to buy gasoline. Business owners approach their paper products, cardboard boxes, and even employee uniforms with the economic principle in mind. So what makes health care any different? Cost is equal to the number of units consumed multiplied by the price at which they were consumed. If health insurance is just health care financing, to lower health insurance costs, we must reduce the number of units of health care we consume or the price at which we consume them. The US health care system does not financially reward those that deliver health care based on outcomes; rather, it rewards those that deliver health care based on the number of health care units they provide. In the same way, our system does not allow consumers to understand the actual cost of health care until after it is delivered, which prevents them from making wise decisions as to where they might receive care. In a free market system, we must provide consumers with access to information and choice so that they can make the right decisions for themselves and move the market appropriately. If you solve the economics of health care, you solve health care. While we will discuss, in the next chapter, the various players in the health care game, we must recognize that some players will not willingly change their methodology, so we will need government intervention. We will also need consumer intervention. Combine a free market system supported by a fair playing field with transparent information, and you will find the solution to health care is not far behind.

CHAPTER 4

Don't Hate the Players; Hate the Game

In today's health care environment, it's easy to make "villains" out of the various players within the system; however, we must remember that, without some of the most vilified pieces within our system (hospital systems, pharmaceutical companies, insurance companies, and so on) and the capitalistic nature in which they tend to operate, we would not have the innovative and impactful system we do today. While many are quick to point fingers and march in protest, those same people might find themselves grateful for these same companies' ingenuity if and when their own health dictates their needing goods and services provided by these parts within the system. That said, we should realize that health care is a game—a game of business—and that if we want to have an impact on how the game is played, we must be aware of it and that if we want to change the game, we must acknowledge the possible consequences.

As we begin thinking through the solutions to our health care woes, we must recognize the structures and incentives by which our current platform operates. From a consumer perspective, health care is often approached like a game of checkers, with each move being made one at a time; however, from an industry perspective, the players are often immersed in a game of chess, thinking many moves ahead. If we, the end users, are to play the game of chess that is health care, we must identify the pieces on the board, their history, and how the various pieces play off of one another to keep the costs (and profits) so high.

They're All Out to Get You

In the past, I often referred to the health care system in the United States as a three-legged stool, with each leg supporting the whole. Within one leg is the delivery system (hospitals, doctors, labs, pharmaceutical companies); within another leg is the finance system (insurance companies); within the final leg is the consumer system (you and me). I no longer refer to the US health care system as the three-legged stool; rather, I refer to it as the three-headed cannibalistic dragon, as both the delivery system and the finance system continue to feed off of one another, and you and I, the consumer, find ourselves at the bottom of the food chain. Over the past decade, we've seen more collaboration within the delivery and finance systems. To see an example of this, we must look no further than the pharmaceutical structure of the delivery system.

Within the United States, all prescription drugs are bought and sold by middle men called pharmacy benefit managers, or PBMs. PBMs are responsible for negotiating drug prices with pharmaceutical companies, then selling those drugs to you and me, all the while using the insurance companies to pick up the tab (only to pass along that cost by way of insurance premiums). Roughly 75 percent of all drugs in the United States are distributed by three PBMs. Today, because of consolidation, all three are now owned by or own insurance companies (Express Scripts and Cigna, Optum and United Healthcare, and, finally, CVS and Aetna). While this is just one example of consolidation, there are multiple others involving labs, hospitals, doctors, and medical device companies. If there is to be a free market system, the consumer must have the power to be the fourth influencer of health care and to set the playing field appropriately—this is where the US Government will come into play (more on this shortly).

The Unwilling Agents of Change

The primary beneficiaries of the US health care system are those that find themselves on either the delivery side or the finance side of health care. In our current structure, these two influencers wield the most power, in large part because, as we'll learn momentarily, the government steers pretty clear of its obligation and role. As such, we, the consumers, end up financing our health care not only via the out-of-pocket dollars we spend on care but also via our insurance premiums or via taxes we pay that go to federal programs such as Medicare and Medicaid.

At the turn of the nineteenth century, the United States experienced the Industrial Revolution. Innovations in manufacturing brought new jobs, opportunity, and wealth. The twentieth century saw an economic shift: wealth was derived more from the buying and selling of things rather than the creating of things. Today, amidst the early twenty-first century, one of the fastest growing sectors of wealth creation can be found in health care and wellness. Diseases and illnesses may not have an economic agenda, but those treating them do.

"More treatment is always better. Default to the most expensive option. A lifetime of treatment is preferable to a cure. Amenities and marketing matter more than good care. As technologies age, prices can rise rather than fall. There is no free choice. Patients are stuck. And they're stuck buying American. More competitors vying for business doesn't mean better prices; it can drive prices up, not down. Economies of scale don't translate to lower prices. With their market power, big providers can simply demand more."

—*Dr. Elizabeth Rosenthal,* An American Sickness

Technology, business, and the American population all grew so fast that legislation and the common citizen were unable to keep up with them. Unlike almost every other industry, the medical industry was in command, instead of the consumer. If you don't like the cost of a product, don't buy it. The prices will drop eventually. But, in an industry where it's literally "buy or die," the consumer doesn't have that choice.

Where Change Can Happen

Since the delivery system and the finance system are not likely going to change their methodology, we must focus our attention on the influencers that can: Uncle Sam and you and me.

The Role of Government

When someone complains that the cost of something is so high because the government is at fault, I usually assume they're wearing a tinfoil hat, and I go my merry way. But, with health care, there is some truth to that complaint. Government's role is, first and foremost, to protect its citizens. Next, to build an infrastructure, and then to set boundaries by which a flourishing society must operate. Yes, I'm referring to rules (also known as regulations). For my conservative friends, the word "regulation" is often one that is met with resistance, but when we are balancing capitalism with care, rules are a must. This is the area where the US government has absolutely failed its citizens. Our government is run by people, and people are easily influenced (not always in the best way). As a result of this influence, combined with a lack of understanding as to how the entire health care system operates, we're left with legislation such as the Medicare Prescription Drug, Improvement, and Modernization Act (MMA), which intended to make drugs less expensive to senior citizens but actually resulted in a massive increase in overall pricing to the general public because of the inefficient way in which the law was drafted. Much like the MMA, the Patient Protection and Affordable Care Act (PPACA)—often called Obamacare—intended to lower the cost of health insurance but actually increased the cost of health care, which is financed by insurance premiums. Thus, insurance premiums have continued to rise. I love that our country tries to help people. I love that people came together and said, "Prescriptions are getting too expensive; we need to help people pay for them," and, "We need to do something about the rise in the cost of health insurance." But where there is a leak, someone will stick a bucket. When you write legislation promising that the US government will buy or subsidize a product (for instance, a prescription through Medicare Part D or a health insurance premium through the ACA), you can be sure that the price of the unit in question will rise as fast as those selling the unit can manage it. The problem with both the MMA and the ACA is that they focused only on one slice of the proverbial pie and set certain rules and regulations without considering the entire platform; as a result, the overall system has become less effective and even less efficient. The government *must* play a role in solving the health care crisis in the United States, but it must do so carefully, so as not to tip the applecart of our free market economy. "Regulation" may be a bad word to some, but, I assure you, no one really wants to drive his or her family down a highway with no speed limits, and, in the same way, the government must set a fair playing field for our health care system to reward ingenuity and effectiveness, while protecting its citizens.

The Consumer

Finally, we've arrived at the real crux of the problem: you and me. Americans have become so disinterested, so locked out and ignored, when it comes to their own health care, which is as intimately personal as it is possible to be, that the industry is allowed to get away with just about anything, because the average consumer has no practical way to fight back and, as a result, has become disengaged as a consumer. While we are culpable in our lack of a consumer's approach to health care, we're not entirely at fault, as it's what we've been accustomed to. Think back to the old movies you watched as a kid: who was often the most trusted advisor in the town? The wise old doctor, of course. Patients had the utmost trust that their doctors were taking care of them to the best of their ability, without thinking about which procedure they could provide that would cost their patients the most. Doctors back then made a decent living, compensated with either goods or money, and the consumers were taken care of—a win-win for everyone. While this plays out well on the big screen and was essentially the way things were "back in the day," the setting has changed. Today, most of us don't know our doctor. We often use an insurance company's website to query the type of provider we're looking for on the basis of our specific insurance network. Once we arrive to a location we've never been before, we fill out a twenty-page legal document that we can't decipher, even if we had a lawyer in our pocket. We then agree to pay our "ultimate debts" (oddly enough, the page for them is usually pretty clear); that's followed by the inevitable waiting and then finally, we're seen by the doctor. The doctors are quick, often disinterested, and regularly act as if their only concern is providing the fastest fix possible before they head off to the other twenty patients in line. We're handed a printout of a five-page diagnosis of our ailment; then we're sent off to either a specialist to treat our condition or to a pharmacy to collect pills of some sort—a drug whose name we usually can't pronounce. At no point, from the time when we step into a doctor's office to the time when we visit a specialist or a pharmacy, do we have any idea what this journey just cost. Does any of this sound familiar? After this fun experience, we Americans often find that, one to three months after services are rendered, we receive what is called an explanation of benefits (an EOB), which doesn't actually explain any of the benefits we received. Soon after the EOB arrives, we receive an invoice from the provider, informing us of the final amount owed. No, not the prices of the individual items, but just a generic, "You owe _____." And herein lies the real problem. In a free market system, the consumer has the power. Want to lower the cost of health care? Allow the consumer to be the consumer. We consumers have immense power, but in today's climate, we don't wield our power. If we did, competition would thrive, goods and services would improve, and the system would work. But when it comes to health care in the United States, the system doesn't work—at least not for those that need it the most.

Even with all the advancements in the freedom of medical information, from services like WebMD to any other number of online websites, we are not doctors. American citizens cannot reliably diagnose what is medically wrong. We rely on others to take care of us, and we are left to hope that when we're told the services cost $20,000, we actually received $20,000 worth of care. It's not our fault. There was no menu board above the receptionist's station, with costs broken down. We didn't know that strep test was going to cost $170, nor, quite frankly, did we really know if we even needed it. In today's system, we are kept from knowing the cost of care and what care is necessary, and that is done quite intentionally. As a result, when it comes to health care, we have become bad consumers, and that's just how the other parties want it.

There Is Hope

Health care is no longer personal in the United States; it is a business. And, unfortunately, it's grown so big that the only way to solve the problems it has caused is to either completely hit the reset button, which isn't feasible, or to install a new set of parameters on it—we can call them regulations.

To continue the metaphor from the beginning of the chapter, each piece on a chessboard is no less vital to winning the game than another. Those of you who play know that one of the worst problems to face is your own pieces blocking your advance; such is the nature of health care. Purposely, health care is obfuscated, made confusing, and made unhelpful. This is done intentionally—to keep your pieces from moving across the board and to keep you from seeing how to win the game.

Hospitals, doctors, big pharma, and insurance companies are *all* necessary in the health care system but none are likely to change. The real solution can be found within two key players on the chessboard: Uncle Sam and us. Yes, government intervention will be required to cure our modern health care system, but so will my intervention and yours.

When I sat down to write this book, my goal was to help change things. Information is power, and I hope we can arrive at a place where common sense prevails and where we get health care back on track to the point where it is consistently accessible and affordable to all people, regardless of their economic status.

The transformative key for consumers is to create a system that is open and honest and transparent and to give them tools and resources to be better consumers. Our health care system can be fixed, and the insanity around it can be stopped, while we maintain economic structure and innovative ingenuity. There are three core principles to solving the problems of health care in the United States:

1. Make health care more transparent.
2. Put the consumer back in the driver's seat.
3. Regulate how health care is delivered from a business perspective.

If we, as a nation, will collectively adhere to these three core principles, it's not going to be that complex for us to get back on track. And if we do so, we, as citizens, can receive the care we need when we need it, new advancements can continue, and those that deliver, finance, and improve health can still make money—good money. It's still a free market system, but now competition can enter into the space more effectively, and the consumer can navigate the competition more efficiently. The solution cannot be applied incrementally; rather, we must tackle all three major components of health care in the United States (the provider, the payer, and the patient) all at the same time.

How does transformation occur? It's only the courageous who are willing to stand up and make waves. For many years, I was part of the problem, but my conscience had a breaking point, and I discovered that I could no longer continue to operate in a method that I knew was not in the best interest of those that were looking to me for advice and counsel, so I chose to expose the system for the way it is. In the same way, will you continue to operate now with the knowledge of how the system works in the same manner in which you have operated in the past? Instead, let us all be an instrument of change and say, "I'm not going to take it anymore!" I can't force you to do one or the other; I can just give you the truth. Health care is a game, and we are one of the players. We must demand that the rules be enforced, and, when necessary, we must demand that new rules be written. We have the power, and it's time we start using it.

CHAPTER 5

The Referee

In any game between players, first, there must be rules by which to play and, second, a referee to ensure the rules are enforced and play is fair. When it comes to the game of health care, however, the rules are limited, and the referee is absent, meaning some players have a more competitive edge. As we begin to think about the government's role in health care, we must acknowledge that our society is as polarized as ever. Health care is among one of the most divisive issues in US politics; however, many health care ideas presented by Democrats have been, at times, supported by Republicans, and vice versa. The support of or opposition to these health care ideas seem to be less about their merit and more about which party is presenting them. Without government intervention at some level, our health care system will not change. As we discussed in the last chapter, it's not as if the corporations within health care are going to voluntarily change their business practices, but at what level should we be comfortable with Uncle Sam's involvement? Should the government be more of a regulatory body or the actual administrator of the system itself?

As we head towards the next set of elections, there have been numerous proposed ideas as to how we should fix health care. These proposed solutions are often based on polarized opinions, most of which are not compatible with the others. This is the nature of health care, which is rarely a small enterprise, and can be a life-and-death issue for some people. It is okay to have a strong opinion on the subject, and we should consider every possible solution, but in our consideration, we should also be calculated and realistic, not naïve. Health care is a behemoth industry in the United States, which fuels a significant portion of the engine of our economy: $1 in $6 is spent on health care. Thus, we must be delicate, indeed, in order to improve what we have, without economic collapse.

Government-Run Health Care

While some on the left believe that we should continue building on the Affordable Care Act, known colloquially as Obamacare, others believe we should move towards a goal called single-payer health care (often referred to as Medicare For All). This system would be similar to those currently found in many of the socialized health care systems throughout Europe. The people who support this idea are very adamant about their position. They eat, sleep, and breathe single-payer. There are variables, of course, within this group; some people feel that government-run health care should cover all health needs, such as long-term care, nursing homes, hearing, dental, and vision. Others with a strong belief in single-payer feel that it should encompass only various combinations of those needs. Regardless, single-payer or Medicare For All would be a drastic restructuring of health care in this country, with the practical effect of making private insurance defunct, or in certain legislative versions, illegal.

The idea of government removing the burden of health care may sound wonderful to some, and there are many who feel that we have a moral obligation to provide health services to every single person who needed it, but the services have to be paid for. And that's the ugly truth of single-payer or Medicare For All: in its current state, there is absolutely no reasonable way to pay for it and still maintain a vibrant economy with an innovative and effective system. According to conservative estimates conducted by numerous agencies, the most recent proposals of single payer or Medicare For All would cost more than $3 trillion per year. That number is too large to be grasped easily. To put that into perspective, the United States military budget (which is often criticized for its size) is about $580 billion per year. That budget is larger than that of China, Russia, Saudi Arabia, India, France, the United Kingdom, and Japan combined, with enough left over to buy every citizen a Starbucks coffee once a day for a month (30 bn+). Currently, the US government's revenue is just over $3 trillion per year. Knowing this, it's a matter of economics. In order to reach the approximate $3 trillion per year to fund single payer we would have to either double tax revenues or take all of the military funding and then use six years of its allocated funding per year just to reach one year for funding. Countries that currently have socialized medicine have tax rates often four times higher than we pay in the US, and while those health care systems are, on the whole, incredibly well-managed, they still struggle to deliver health care in a timely and efficient manner to their citizens, many times rationing care because of a lack of funding or resources.

Funding isn't the only issue. The US government's infrastructure is neither currently capable nor effective enough to manage the behemoth of health care, which I can prove to you with two specific examples. The first is a government-run health care system our government provides—Veterans Affairs. All of the foibles and failings of the VA that we have watched play out in the media of late have been the result of the government's inability to manage health care from a business perspective. It's simply not equipped to do it. I heard it once said by a veteran receiving benefits from the VA that it was like "giving veterans a second chance to die for their country." Diving deeper into the failings of the VA, on August 31, the Friday before Labor Day 2018, at 4:56p.m., the Department of Veteran's affairs released its report, as it was obligated to do under the VA MISSION Act of 2018. I note the time, because it's often the period news reporters refer to as "dumping it with the trash" (a reference to releasing information you really don't want people to know). On that particular day, it was reported that there were currently 45,239 job vacancies at the Department of Veteran Affairs, resulting in an 11 percent staffing gap. Think of where you work and how effective your company would be if one in ten of your coworkers just stood up and walked away. Furthermore, in March 2010, an internal VA audit showed that one in four disability claims had errors. Care is often denied because of these errors, and the average claim takes nearly four months to be processed. At the current time of writing this book, the VA has nearly 340,000 claims pending in its backlog. Is this how one could expect government-run health care to operate?

Another example of the potential effectiveness in a government-run health care system and how it might operate can be found in how we travel in the United States. If you've flown in the past decade, you've experienced the joy that is the TSA. This is an organization that was designed from the ground up by the US government in the days following the terrorist attacks of September 11, 2001. No expense was spared, and yet, with the best and brightest minds of the federal government designing a system to keep us safe, the TSA has a 95 percent failure rate for detecting weapons and contraband. That bears repeating—one out of twenty times, the TSA employees succeed in doing their jobs. And is this the type of administration people think should dictate our health care, determining whether we need certain tests to detect cancer and other life-threatening diseases?

Beyond the sheer cost and the unlikely chance that a government-run health care system would be designed to function well, the sheer economic damage a single-payer system would create would be devastating. Consider the number of jobs that would be lost. Single payer or Medicare For All would make most of the people in the insurance industry superfluous. Currently employed in health insurance and its ancillary parts are approximately 3 million Americans. Once you factor in indirect supporting positions, such as custodial services, technical services, food services, administrative services, call centers, and so on, that number is closer to about 5 million employees. Some have said it's a matter of principle, but for those in the real world, we recognize that it's a matter of economics. Sure, we may want to clothe all of the children of the world, but we only have so much cloth, and wishing won't make it so. We must be realistic.

Free Market Capitalism Run Amuck

On the opposite end of the "Medicare For All" or "single-payer" camp can be found the often more conservative crowd. On the whole, many in this group believe that the way things are going right now (or, more specifically, prior to the ACA) are fine and that we should simply maintain the status quo and allow the market to take care of itself. The issue with this thinking is that maintaining the status quo or returning to a pre-ACA world is equally untenable and that when it comes to health care, our free market system doesn't work the way it does in other areas of our economy. Health care costs are out of control and are increasing at a rate unmatched by inflation or wage growth. Because of a lack of proper transparency, the current "free market" isn't working either, but it could. In a proper market, consumers have the tools at their disposal to make confident, informed purchasing decisions, even on complicated issues.

Regulated Free Market

As stated earlier, the United States is responsible for the vast majority of innovation when it comes to health care, and it is this innovation that supports the more socialized systems throughout the world. Other nations can have socialized medicine, because we don't here in the United States. But we must be able to maintain our free market ingenuity, while allowing our free market to control cost. This works in every other aspect of our system, because we have a regulated free market, where the government requires truth in pricing and transparency and allows for open competition.

> **Example:** I want to buy a toaster. One store has the toaster advertised for $20, while the other has it advertised for $45. More people will buy the less expensive unit, and sales of that cheaper toaster go through the roof. While the cheaper price may be raised slightly, because of demand, at the same time, the more expensive unit either lowers its price or develops an improved product to justify its additional cost. Sales begin to even out between the two models, and new products will come to market to compete.

In this scenario, the market has functioned as intended, with the consumer able to compare prices, qualities of the units, and then make personal decisions on the basis of what they want. This is how almost everything in our economy works: houses, cars, consumer goods, luxury items, and so forth—but not health care. When it comes to the health care industry, prices and options are hidden behind years of corporate lobbying, while having secured those companies very favorable laws and advantages over the American consumer, thus denying the market's ability to fluctuate up and down in a manner that benefits the consumer. This is what needs to change.

It's said that sunlight is the best disinfectant and that things done in the dark should always be brought to light. The lack of transparency is the number-one driver of the exorbitant prices and increases we pay each year. Outside influence notwithstanding, it's not likely that particular pharmaceutical companies, hospital systems, or health insurers will wake up one day and decide they are making too much money. While some businesses might serve a noble purpose, most share both a primary and fiduciary obligation to return a level of profit to their shareholders as high as possible.

A well-intentioned, but fairly naïve, response would be to suggest that we require all hospitals and health insurers to be nonprofit, but the specific tax status of an organization doesn't necessarily change its objective. I've walked through many nonprofit hospitals, with marble floors and expensive artwork, and I've known plenty of nonprofit insurers with seven-figure executive compensation structures. A nonprofit system would just ensure that all profits are properly liquidated. Remember that the NFL is a nonprofit company, too, and I've seen how much their Superbowl commercials cost. Every organization delivering health care is actually for-profit; their official tax status does not make it otherwise. Prices will not lower, or at least stop climbing at such prodigious rates, unless outside pressure is brought to bear on these companies through a combination of both competition and regulation.

We must require specific parameters surrounding multiple areas of our current system. Medical billing, insurance networks, unnecessary tests and procedures, tort reform, how patents are procured and extended, new drugs brought to market, fee-for-service invoicing, in-and-out-of-network procedures, and many other areas are all things the US government should set parameters surrounding them or, at the very least, provide for consumer beneficial transparency. In the remaining chapters, we will outline specific measures that can be taken to address each of these areas. Some will require government intervention, and some will require consumer engagement. Either way, solutions will be outlined.

To those on the left who read this chapter with frustration, I understand. But as frustrating as it is to hear and just as easy as it is to hand-wave away with, "We'll increase taxes; we'll find the money," single-payer insurance will not work until a series of problems can be overcome, chiefly monetary, with competence and design just behind.

To those on the right who believe we must keep government out of health care, I, too, believe we should have limited government involvement, but at the same time, I recognize that, without government influence, costs will continue to rise, and the consumer will not be provided with the ability to effectively navigate and influence the system, thus eliminating the true nature of a free market system.

Don't give up, yet.

Each of these pieces—the delivery system, the finance system of insurance, and the consumer system—will play a key role in solving health care, but the lynchpin is Uncle Sam. The US government must step in to better set the rules of the game in a way that makes it fair to all parties. In a free market, there is transparency, and with transparency, progress.

CHAPTER 6

The Doctor Will See You Now

"The doctor will see you now" is a phrase we don't regularly hear anymore; instead, in today's health care environment, it's more along the lines of having a 10:00 a.m. appointment, which you show up for at 9:45, fill out miles of paperwork, wait till 10:20, be taken back to a room, asked questions by a nurse, wait twenty more minutes, spend five actual minutes with the doctor, and receive a bill for $200 next month. In today's health care environment, a routine visit to see a doctor feels more like speed dating than it does time spent with a trusted advisor.

Time and Money

Today, specifically for physicians, time is literally money. Many doctors are under increased time constraints, as insurers are paying them less, but countering the reduced pay by sending doctors' offices a large volume of patients instead.[1] The result is both unhappy patients and unhappy doctors, each fighting for time that they both deserve.

So how did we get here and what was the cause of this? Journey with me to the distant year of 1992, where Disney's *Aladdin* was released, the computer game Oregon Trail was all the rage, and Medicare adopted the relative value unit (RVU) as the standard formula by which to calculate doctor's fees.[2] On the basis of this methodology, an average physician's office visit should be 1.3 RVUs, which, using the American Medical Association (AMA) coding guidelines, equates to approximately fifteen minutes. And there you have it, a guideline for restricting time. Who would have known that the same year that brought us the Mall of America, NAFTA, and "I didn't inhale" would be the same year that has caused significant damage between the relationships of doctors and their patients. The actual formula (RVU x Geographic Index + Practice Expenses RVU + Liability Insurance RVU x Medicare Conversion Factor) is assessed, in conjunction with the Center for Medicare and Medicaid Services (CMS) every five years,[3] but the assessment itself isn't intended to address the issue of delivering proper care; rather, it is updated to more accurately determine the costs for the physician's services. As a result, the 1.3 RVU value hasn't changed, meaning fifteen minutes is still the established standard time for an "average" doctors' visit today.

While the expected time spent with a doctor has not changed in nearly thirty years, what has changed is the amount of time that same physician must spend on paperwork he or she is expected to file in regard to each visit. Over the years, as more technology has been introduced and electronic health records were created to theoretically increase the expediency in the sharing of information between providers, the end result is that more time is spent by doctors doing data entry and less time interacting with the patient themselves. In a study published in the *Annals of Internal Medicine*, doctors are unable to use the full fifteen minutes talking to or examining patients. While in the examining room, doctors are spending approximately half of their time (52.9 percent), interacting with the patient and just over a third of their time (37 percent) filling out paperwork. Where has the other 10 percent gone, you might ask? That question leads us to another problem in today's health care environment. Since fifteen minutes is the recommended time for each patient, business-run practices, hospital systems, and clinics often demand that doctors see four patients per hour (fifteen minutes x four patients = one hour). While that math may work per the RVU guidelines, what doesn't add up is that this allotment of time does not allow for transit between rooms, needing to consult with nurses, printing out necessary forms, writing prescriptions, or even doing human things, like taking a restroom break. All of those necessary acts are not calculated into the allotted time; thus the added minutes needed for these things are generated by reducing time spent with the patient, who, as a result, is now reduced to less than an average of eight minutes of actual consultative time with the doctor. With the average billing cost of $200 for a walk-in clinic appointment, a patient being billed $25 per minute has become a tough pill to swallow, not to mention a decline in the engagement of long-term care between a patient and the doctor. With limited time and multiple patients to see, the doctor is left to either refer a patient to a specialist or to prescribe a pill rather than developing a relationship with someone whose health and care they can truly influence.

The impersonal impact of the limited time with doctors has led to a rise in what we will refer to as "ill-advised consumerism." Patients' responses to the combination of lack of meaningful time and long waits for appointments with their doctors, coupled with the prohibitive costs associated with what end up often being multiple visits for the same issue, have led to patients either self-diagnosing via the internet or conversationally with people they know or, even worse, not going to see a physician at all. Today's lack of proper engagement with a primary care physician has, according to many studies, led to roughly half of the US population skipping out on recommended annual exams. These challenges have transitioned the relationship of patient and doctor from that of a trusted advisor to one of conflict between the two parties. I've personally seen in the administrative wing of doctors' offices signs that read, "Don't mistake your Google search with my medical degree." While this may seem like a clever quote, more important, it indicates a dismissive attitude that many doctors have to being questioned or second-guessed. Doctors are no longer seen as ones with whom to seek counsel, but rather an avenue to treatment. In today's ill-advised, consumeristic world, patients are more apt to arrive at their doctor's offices with a self-diagnosis and predetermined preferred treatment regimen based on time spent on WebMD or some other search engine. As a result, when a doctor either arrives at a different diagnosis or selects an alternative form of treatment than the patient had expected on the basis of his or her own research, there is conflict and thus poor adherence to the prescribed course from the doctor.[4]

Furthermore, doctors' approaches under severe time constraints can lead to preventable errors. Like all others, doctors are people and can fall into patterns or jump to conclusions too early. It's easy to see the same batch of symptoms and to prescribe a "one-size-fits-all" antibiotic, when specific care tailored to the specific ailment would be better suited. Both parties want what is the best for the patient, but they are at loggerheads as to how to achieve it.

This is one of the easiest fixes you'll read about in this book, yet it may prove to be one of the hardest to implement. We must change the RVU formula to allow doctors greater time with their patients.

It's that simple. By doing this, we alleviate numerous struggles within the industry and increase the possibility of improved health. More time with the patient leads to more accurate diagnoses and a stronger bond with the doctor, which then leads to a higher likelihood that what is prescribed as treatment would be followed. While the patient would agree to this change wholeheartedly, the business-minded doctor and the insurer are not as likely to encourage this change. Primary care physicians (PCPs) traditionally do not perform procedures or surgeries, which are the big-ticket items for generating large volumes of revenue. Instead, PCPs are most often paid per visit, with only slight adjustments for interactions that run longer. Remember that profits are also about the number of units distributed. In our current fee-for-service system, more time with the patients would lead to fewer patients being seen, which, in turn, leads to fewer profits for the practice, the hospital system, or the clinic.

I'm not advocating that providers be unfairly compensated for their work; rather, the beauty of the free market, if not constrained, is that it will adapt to changing circumstances. We needn't look any further than the recent emergence of the concierge clinic, where, in exchange for a monthly membership fee, patients have exclusive access to certain practitioners, with easily available appointments as often and as regularly as they are needed. These concierge services often also include patient advocacy teams, which connect with outside specialists, hospitals, and other health providers on behalf of their members to find higher-quality treatment at a lower cost when necessary. This leads to a better patient-and-doctor relationship,[5] as the patients' care is truly directed by a primary care doctor who has developed a relationship with the patient.

As it stands today, the United States is experiencing a growing shortage of general practitioners. Current research estimates we will have a shortage of at least 42,600 to as high as 121,300 primary care physicians by the year 2030.[6] This is concerning, given that currently more than 66 million Americans live in health professional shortage areas or areas where the ratio of general care providers to citizens is deemed insufficient by the federal government. Compounding that issue even further is that people are living longer; baby boomers are living longer lives and are subject to more complex illnesses and comorbidities than before.[7] Cancer, arthritis, cardiac diseases, and diabetes are all common conditions among the elderly, which require a moderate to significant amount of care. This issue of longevity is then multiplied by the increased coverages afforded through the Affordable Care Act, which is projected to need an additional 17,000 doctors than would have been needed without it.[8] Access to more care increases the demand for it, and a Gallup poll shows that people are indeed using it.[9] Continuing fears that the ACA might be overturned or legislatively eliminated are causing more Americans to utilize their health care while they can.[10]

The solution to this is twofold. First, we must increase the number of general practitioners we have, and we must better allocate physicians and their resources throughout the country. Both are easier said than done. Training new doctors is not an overnight process—it takes between twelve and fifteen years' worth of education and training after high school to become a licensed physician, so any solutions that we implement now will take nearly a decade and a half to bear fruit. Beyond this, the process for the number of residency programs is complicated.

There currently exists a cap on the number of new doctors allowed to be trained each year in the United States: 28,000. One would think that, clearly, we need to remove the cap and allow more doctors to work, thereby diminishing the shortage; however, the United States only produced around 19,000 new medical graduates last year, and many of these move into specialty practices rather than general medicine (in large part because of the potential income). Fortunately, we're able to shore up the remaining spots with doctors who were trained in accredited programs in foreign countries. Our problems are not due to a lack of medical schools. Since 2002, the United States has had thirteen new medical schools open—an increase of about 10 percent. Concurrently, the number of med school graduates has risen from 15.5 thousand to 19 thousand. This closely mirrors the overall population growth of the United States. The shortage of doctors, specifically primary care physicians or general practitioners, is primarily the result of cost. While many more of our students may feel led to work in health care, the high cost can be destructive and prohibitive. The average graduate of medical school carries more than $200,000 in debt, with more than 25 percent of students graduating with over than $300,000[11] in debt. The United States needs more general practitioners, but the overwhelming debt for those willing to bear the cost leads them into other areas of medicine—specialties.

Cost and opportunity for profit are driving our doctors into specialty practices. How else would a young physician plan to pay off a half million of debt? Our shortage problem is a shortage of general practitioners, not specialists. In the United States, only around 30 percent of physicians are general practitioners, with the remaining 70 percent varying in some form of specialists (—ologists).[12] The gatekeeper to better health is the primary care physician. Only when things go wrong do Americans most often utilize the services of a specialist. Approximately one in five Americans had an appointment with a specialist doctor[13] in 2016, with half of those appointments for a primary care issue and not requiring specialization.[14] That math comes out to being nine out of ten times we need a PCP, not an specialist. While this situation is dire to the American consumer, it's a perfect storm for the business-led hospital system and pharmaceutical industry, who utilize today's PCPs as the sales force to either prescribe a pill or refer to a higher-cost specialist.

Plain and simple, we need more PCPs, which would require making access to medical school more affordable. Don't get me wrong here. I'm not advocating making medical school itself any easier; it should be one of the most rigorous and intensive areas of study imaginable. Becoming a doctor should require exceptional minds, uncommon fortitude, and mental strength beyond the common person. When you wield the power of life and death over your patients within your mind and the tools in your hands, I want it to be exceptionally difficult to graduate from medical school. After all, I may be on your operating table someday. But, for those who possess those qualities, the inability to pay the upfront cost should not be the barrier to entry. The solution, then, is to make medical school more affordable.

In 2018, NYU Medical School did something absolutely brazen—they made it free. They received enough in donations to sustain this practice for the foreseeable future. If you could pass the entry exams, your tuition was paid for, upfront, in its entirety. The vitriol this caused was a level of toxicity rarely seen. Articles made comments like, "*What a waste. An expensive, unnecessary subsidy for elite medical grads who stand to make a killing.*"[15] It's easy to think that anyone who goes to medical school must come from a rich family, as, historically, that is oftentimes what it *has* taken. It's easy to continue to assume that this is just the rich perpetuating that cycle, but the data says otherwise.

NYU Med saw a 102 percent increase in applications from those who are members of a group underrepresented in medicine, those being black, Latino, and American Indian. The largest percentage of increase (142 percent) came from those who identify as black, Afro-Caribbean, or African American.[16] An important detail to remember is that qualifying for medical school is no easy task. One has to take the MCAT, a rigorous test similar to the SATs (but on steroids), plus the requisite courses in high school, such as biology, anatomy and physiology, organic chemistry (essentially any course that would have made me rip my hair out and run out the door). These students are not applying "just" because tuition became free; they already had the chops to become doctors, and the primary factor stopping them was cost. We have those exceptional minds within our society; we just need to make the door more accessible to walk through.

Again, the issue of having too many specialists and not enough general practitioners is the price of admission. A study of 124 medical schools, with a combination of both private and public institutions, found disturbing data on this front. Students with high debt relative to that of their peers at their home institution reported "*higher frequencies of feeling callous towards others, were more likely to choose a specialty with a higher average annual income, were less likely to plan to practice in underserved locations, and were less likely to choose primary care.*"[17] These are young adults, barely old enough to drink, yet they are making choices about financial decisions larger than most mortgages that will affect them for just as long. This survey also finds that these students will most likely delay getting married, delay buying a house, report higher levels of depression and stress related to their finances, and significantly worry that the choice of their education will influence the choice of their medical field.

None of what I have written above should be taken as a cry for the financial plight of doctors in general; they are still more likely than any other profession to be in the top 1 percent of earners, but it is important to recognize that there are financial drivers at play and that they do affect the career choice of the medical student. Over the course of their career, the average general practitioners will reach an income level of $189,000 per year—but not when they start practicing. It takes doctors nearly ten years after their residency to reach the median earning levels of their peers. While in their starting years as residents, the average annual income is $55,400 per year.[18] When you split the difference and see that the average resident works sixty-five hours per week, the rate of pay equates to $16.39 per hour, or less than most food-service managers. While a primary care physician might eventually hit that average $189,000 income, this still pales in comparison to an orthopedic surgeon's average $519,000 annual paycheck, a cardiologist's average $512,000 annual paycheck, and a urologist's average $461,000 annual paycheck.[19] If, for the same relative years of training and effort, a young physician can choose a career that will net an additional $6 million over the course of a working career of thirty years, we can see that would be a very tempting choice for many.[20]

There's an argument to be made, certainly, that it's not the responsibility of the federal government to train new doctors, and I'm not advocating for free college, but for the moment, let's set that aside. Let us instead look at the larger picture. We have a growing and critical shortage of doctors in rural areas. We need to expand access to primary care, which, in turn, if done appropriately, would curb the long-term cost of chronic conditions that are likely going unnoticed or improperly treated early on. Preventative medicine and early-onset treatment is much less expensive than care for major conditions that could have been prevented or, at the very least, identified early on, but all too often, patients are not getting the proper counsel they so desperately need because the time is simply not available. While this leads to decreased health, it, in turn, leads to increased profits, as the treatment and care for these major issues generates significant income for the medical system. We have programs in place that have helped alleviate these shortages, but they need to be expanded at the state level. The National Health Service Corps (NHSC) is a federal program that helps physicians and medical students with student-loan-debt relief in exchange for service in underserved areas. There are currently 10,200 NHSC doctors at work, with another 1,400 in training.[21] In the 2018 fiscal year, several thousand applicants were turned away, because the allocated funding was spent.[22]

Needless to say, there's much more to be done here, and unfortunately, without government intervention, we will likely move forward with little to no change. There's no easy solution to this problem, but we must, as a society, begin to realize our problem and work together to solve it. More PCPs leads to better care, which leads to lower cost—remember that it's the economic principal: to lower the cost, one option is to reduce the number of units consumed. More PCPs in our society will help us achieve this.

CHAPTER 7

Hospitals—America's New "Too Big to Fail"

I'm sure you're familiar with the Hippocratic oath; it's the ethical foundation of the entire medical profession, upon which physicians build their careers. Hippocrates' oath contained a long paragraph that asked medical professionals to swear to do the best they could, to admit the times when they were wrong, to teach their fellow man, and to help people live healthy lives. The oath was abbreviated to its most important tenet a few centuries later—"primum non nocere: first, do no harm." Hospitals were to be places of healing, full of caring, moral individuals, who had made a life out of alleviating suffering.

Ask most doctors why they chose the medical profession, and many will tell you that they wanted to help people. Sure, once they achieve tenure, the income is good, but doctors, especially those starting off, work grueling hours in one of the most stressful jobs in the world, because they can do good for others. Their grueling work is for the betterment of their fellow man and deeply satisfying when done right. This makes it all the worse that a doctor's temple, the hospital, has been corrupted by the exploiters of capitalism. While physicians may still adhere to the Hippocratic oath, many who lead the business side of health care and who are now running many hospital systems live by a different oath—make money for the shareholders. This is dangerous, because while the doctor may be the gatekeeper to the health care system, the hospital is the gateway. It is the conduit to an entire economic system, which sets the parameters for patient care and recovery. Hospitals are the gold standard for treatment and diagnosis, and the doctor who staffs a hospital offers advice and counsel that is beyond contestation. This creates a very dangerous clash, a conflict between capitalism and care.

The current structure and methodology surrounding today's hospital system have not always operated in the manner it did a century ago, or even a generation ago. So how did we find ourselves so far afield from the engaged doctor and charitable hospital? Follow the money, of course. A short history lesson: a generation ago, we knew our banker. We knew the bank. We knew the people on the board of the bank, who were local community folks, people who were from their local region and who invested in it. The betterment of the community drove the economic motivation behind their business decisions. They wanted to see the community thrive and become prosperous. If their peers did well, they did well. It was important that the bank did well financially, of course, to protect from future losses, but people weren't nickel-and-dimed for every transaction. Fast forward to 2008, and the United States found itself engrained in an economic crisis surrounding the banking system: large banks had become even larger by buying up and gobbling up the smaller banks. If they had been towering and faceless before, they were gargantuan and completely opaque entities now.

There would be no peeking behind the curtain. Fee-for-service models were a regular part of the banking system by 2008, and what was once the personal aspect of the community bank had disappeared, replaced by video screens and institutions without tellers. The level of hospitality and service that had been provided in years past became a fond memory in the new era of efficiency.

Market share was gone in the banking industry, as there was little left to be shared. The big conglomerates had bought their way in, and now decisions that had been previously made by community leaders invested in local businesses were instead made by shrewd businesspeople on Wall Street. These new orchestrators of the banking industry people would never see the good or ill their decisions were having on the community that was going to be impacted; they saw only the dollar signs at the bottom of their profit-and-loss statements.

And then, just as it had begun, it ended. The banks had become too greedy and too leveraged, and when their bubble burst, these massive entities didn't have the liquidity to sustain themselves. As the stock market tanked in the aftermath and countless lives were ruined, the only solution was for the US government to step in and stop the bleeding. While many experienced financial ruin, the bankers themselves were given a lifeline, and a new phrase emerged: "too big to fail."

While there have been some changes to the US banking system as a result of the events of 2008, today it is the hospital systems that mirror a business practice similar to that of yesterday's banking system. The once-private practitioner has been folded into a practice. That practice has been replaced by a clinic, and that clinic is now owned by a hospital. And like the banking industry, the consumer has become a number on a page and a dollar sign at the bottom of an invoice. Rinse, and repeat.

In 2012, only 14 percent of physician's practices were owned by hospitals; in 2018, that number is a staggering 68 percent,[23] with no signs of slowing down. Only one-third of doctors surveyed in the 2018 Survey of America's Physicians are now private-practice owners or partners, with almost one half (49.1 percent) identifying as hospital- or medical-group employees.[24] The idea of a hospital system becoming "too big to fail" is approaching rapidly, if it isn't here already.

As such, we can no longer allow hospital systems to be left to their own devices. If they were self-policing, we wouldn't need to be having this conversation. So how do we solve that? How can we create a structure where hospitals can't own the entire market—both the gateway and the gatekeeper? Fortunately for us, that system is already in place. It just needs some minor tweaking, and of course, actual enforcement. We have the FTC (Federal Trade Commission), and the Bureau of Consumer Protection, which exist to enforce antitrust laws, in conjunction with the Department of Justice. However, alas, they clearly haven't been pulling their weight, either. If they had, the checks-and-balances system of the market would have worked. I'm a free market capitalist, and I don't think that there should be a limit as to how successful your business can be, but monopolies are real, and we are seeing them continue to develop with the current hospital system.

To both quantify and prevent monopolies, we have the Herfindahl-Hirschman Index (which we will refer to as the HHI, because Herfindahl-Hirschman Index is too much to say). The HHI is a formula used by the FTC to determine market competitiveness, both pre- and post-M&A transactions. The closer to a monopoly a firm holds, the higher the HHI score will be. It would stand to reason that, above a certain score, a hospital merger would not be allowed to take place. However, hospitals, specifically those that are filed as not-for-profit, have a curious quality—they are first viewed not as a business but as a community resource and a social institution. Thus, we find ourselves within the battle of public perception, as well as market control. To hear it said by the industry itself, Torrey McLary, a lawyer at King & Spalding who specializes in hospital mergers, says that mergers "*can fix a hospital and benefit the community.*"[25] And with that sentiment, these mergers are often approved, because the hospitals are able to make such compelling cases as to how coordinating care and utilizing the economies of scale will reduce costs for the community by 15 percent to 30 percent.[26] The case is also made that, following a merger, smaller hospitals will have access to more capital and thus will be able to make major upgrades to the facilities and investments in new technologies, thereby enhancing efficiency and efficacy of treatments. In response to such positive imagery, courts will ignore their instincts and the HHI score and approve mergers and acquisitions that would have been denied otherwise.[27]

Unfortunately, these courts are looking through rose-tinted glass. According to Zach Cooper, a health economist at Yale University, there is "*near unanimity*"[28] among the academic community that hospital consolidation is driving up health care costs, and the data backs him up, too. A 2018 analysis from the Nicholas C. Petris Center of the University of California-Berkeley found that consolidation consistently leads to higher prices. Analyzing twenty-five metropolitan areas, the center found that the average price for a hospital stay has actually increased from 11 percent to as much as 54 percent,[29] with an average price of hospital services increasing 6 percent to 18 percent.[30] This is not new research; this has been confirmed by the American Health Association (AHA) annual survey, which studied the years from 1985 through 1997, showing a 40 percent increase in hospital prices post-merger,[31] and Capps and Dranove found an 18 percent average increase between 1998 and 2000.[32] These are not small sample sizes; the PricewaterhouseCoopers research spanned over 5,600 individual facilities and 526 health care systems nationwide. Nor was all of this data too narrow in scope. Utilizing CMS data, the research was adjusted to accommodate the geographic disparity in wages and costs, including variables such as number of beds, lengths of stay, full-time-employees per bed, operating margins, and number of admissions.

Hospitals will make a counterargument that technology marches on—in the past thirty years, we have had technological leaps and bounds, and both the training and the equipment are incredibly expensive. While it is fair to allocate higher prices associated with technology, the argument is without merit, as the additional expense should have been accounted for in the M&A approval process within the 15 percent to 20 percent savings that were to occur. While there may be an argument that consolidating does save the hospitals money, that doesn't mean they'll be passing that on to you. Remember: they are businesses.

Regarding the claims that concentrated markets do not correspond to higher costs and that mergers are a great thing for local communities, in a study by Berkeley health economist James Robinson, using data from sixty-one different hospitals and using the HHI formula, it was found that hospitals in concentrated markets, with above-average HHI, charge 44 percent higher prices than hospitals with below-average HHI, even though the two hospital groups had a difference of only 6 percent in operating costs.

To summarize: these are not surveys and reports that are too narrow in scope; they have spanned thousands of hospitals and hundreds of marketplaces. This is not information that is out of date or that does not cover a long-enough period; these reports provide trends that span more than thirty years. These are reliable, accredited sources, including organizations such as PricewaterhouseCoopers, as well as the federal government (CMS and FTC). All of this data proves that too much hospital consolidation is occurring, that it is accelerating, and that it significantly contributes to higher costs.

Since disassembling a merged hospital network would be akin to unscrambling an egg (i.e., impossible), our next step would be to introduce more competition into the markets. Make no mistake; this is definitely the pound of cure, whereas preventing unnecessary mergers is the ounce of prevention. Since that is no longer an option, we must to do the next best thing. In any system, there are several immediate steps that can be taken that would have significant and immediate impact on the competition levels within the markets.

As I have stated numerous times and will do so again, we do not need the government to run health care. We need the government to *regulate* health care. I don't buy into the idea that health care is a "right"; rather, it is a necessity. Part of a society where you have more than one person requires that there be *rules.* If it was just I in the world, there would be no need for such rules, but as soon as it's you and I, there is a need for rules. We must set up parameters and have boundaries in which to conduct fair business. In a society with more than three hundred *million* people, there must be regulatory structures.

We wouldn't want a highway system where drivers could drive at any speed they wish, nor do we want a society where people could do harm to others without any fear of consequences. The challenge we have in health care is that while we may not be seeing a place where we witness violent criminal acts, we do witness a societal criminal act. Unregulated health care systems can operate in a manner that they see fit to reward their investors and their executives and not what is in the best interest of the people that come to them for care, and that's where we need Uncle Sam to step in. In a free market system, the consumer can impact this practice, but, with today's consolidation, we no longer have free market competition and choice. In the absence of transparent competition, we need Uncle Sam to set the boundaries and the parameters. The independent community and state-based boards should pose the question: "What is in the best interest of this community?"

To pose that question, we need to change the scope of the issue. Currently, antitrust and monopolization is observed from the federal level, more of a birds-eye view. But for the average citizen, health care is local. Except for the rare accident while traveling or the need for specialized care elsewhere in the country, most citizens stay within a county or two to receive care. If the health care markets are local, much of the regulation should happen at the local level as well. While the federal government may have good intentions, there can be a dangerous precedent created when the government attempts to define locality from Washington. In the *United States v. Mercy Health Services*,[33] the courts defined the geographic market of Poplar Bluff, Missouri, to include hospitals seventy to one hundred miles away. In *United States v. Carilion Health Services*,[34] the primary market was upheld by the court to included services within a sixteen-county area surrounding Roanoke, Virginia. The sheer scale of those markets, if it were applied to a place like New York City, means that it's "market" could include hospitals in five other states, (Massachusetts, Connecticut, New Jersey, and Delaware). The precedent of those cases renders the ability for a hospital to say it has plenty of competition in a market, even though that market may be encompassing completely different towns and cities, or even states. While it may be legal in a free market system, it's certainly not fair.

First, let's establish what a local market is, and should be. For the people living in Dallas, Texas, which averages approximately twenty miles in diameter, if they should live in the center of town, the edge of the city is about ten miles away in any given direction. But Dallas is a metropolis, with suburbs, rural areas, and medical specialists in various but relatively nearby cities, so limiting a marketplace to a city doesn't work. The parameter could extend to encompass a county, because not all people live in the city's center; some folks would live right on the edge of the city. If the marketplace for a hospital area was defined as the largest distance between the county it resides in and the county next to it, we would see, on average, a diameter of sixty miles diameter, or a half-hour drive in any direction without traffic. While allowing for an exception process for incredibly sparse rural areas, establishing a thirty-mile radius as a hospital marketplace would increase the HHI score, providing a more realistic view of the concentration for preventing the monopolization of the health care market and, at the same time, for preventing hospitals from watering down their HHI scores. There are, of course, other ways to quantify, be it population density, the size of the hospital, and so on, but the point is there is no standard at this time beyond market share, and that clearly hasn't been an accurate determinant.

Now that we've established what a market should be, let's talk about those who can get into that market and the places where the competition has gone. Certificate-of-need (CON) laws are the industry standard for good intentions leading to creating the very thing that health care facilities were trying to prevent. CON laws were originally introduced back in 1974 as part of the Health Planning Resources Development Act. This act was intended to restrain too many health care facilities from opening in a single geographic area. The underlying assumption of CON regulation was that excess capacity from building too many health care facilities would result in higher prices. If hospitals had empty beds and fixed costs had to be paid for, they would raise their prices to make sure they stayed solvent. Ergo, limit the number of hospitals. But it's not just hospitals: while each state has different requirements, the base statutes of CONs include any health care facility.

Hospitals are masters of vertical integration, and for good reason. Hospitals should provide a plethora of medical specialties, as various needs will be met within them. Vertical integration is not only a good business practice; it also provides hospitals with the ability to deliver great medical treatment. We want hospitals to have imaging services, blood labs, genetic testing, and neurology centers. We would like to have every specialist that exists available within hospitals in which we may be seeking care. While, in general, vertical integration benefits patients from a care perspective and hospitals from a business perspective, it can be damaging from a consumer perspective. There needs to be exterior competition from independent practices, but those cannot open without CON approval. In a free market, the ability to oversaturate must be allowed, even to a community's temporary detriment. The market will balance itself out eventually. CON laws exist as protectionism for hospitals, because they are too great a community asset to be allowed to go under. They are, finally, proven to be "Too Big To Fail." According to the George Mason University's Mercatus Center, CON programs are associated with few hospitals in rural and suburban areas,[35] so, by protecting already established hospitals, we are denying other areas their own. The research shows that these exist as only costly barriers of a bygone era to entry for new health care providers rather than useful tools of controlling or improving health care quality.

This is such an obvious case of protectionism by lobbying groups that, in a rare twist, repeal of CON laws are favored by leaders of both political parties. President Obama supported a repeal of CON laws, as does the United States Department of Health and Human Services (HHS) under the Trump Administration.[36,37] As of 2019, fifteen states have successfully repealed their CON programs, and we can only hope that trend continues.

To summarize, hospitals have become "too big to fail," and as my West Texas father would say, "It's hard to put toothpaste back in the tube." That said, while too much consolidation has already occurred, we must halt the practice of future consolidation. If all of the steps outlined within this chapter could happen, would it completely solve the high costs of hospitals and medical billing? No, but they will certainly help, and any percentage of cost you can save in a 3.5 trillion-dollar-per-year industry is worth its weight in gold. We've addressed issues of monopolies in their geographic, legislative, monetary, and intellectual forms. Starting with these basic guidelines will encourage better rules and legislation in the future, as the guardrails will be in place to help keep the hospitals in check and on track and hopefully help you be a better consumer. As is the constant theme within each of the solutions outlined throughout this book, we must require transparency. In a free market system, the consumer can move the market—we must require the business practices of the hospital system to become more transparent. As health care costs continue to rise, we must begin the turn the tide before we find ourselves in another 2008-like bailout.

CHAPTER 8

Your Money or Your Life

Have you ever received a shocking hospital bill or late fees because of an overdue medical invoice? Most people have.

I'll never forget the first time I really looked at a hospital bill; I had already been working in the health insurance industry for many years, but up until this point, health care had not had a personal impact on my adult life, so my studies of health care billing were detached and clinical. This particular bill, however, arrived after my wife had to undergo a procedure to remove two very large cysts on her ovaries. These cysts had caused extreme pain as well as potential threats to our ability to have children. In an effort to remove the cysts while trying to preserve my wife's ovaries, her OB-GYN would utilize the latest and greatest in robotic technology, and, because of that, the surgery would be extensive and would therefore be performed in a hospital. Even though the surgery was extensive, we would likely be discharged after just a few hours of recovery and observation following the procedure.

Before my wife was rolled back to the operating room, I recall the doctor walking me through the aspects of the procedure. It all seemed very systematic and routine until we got to the end of the description, when the physician stated that I would need to prepare myself should they discover that the ovaries were beyond repair and thus needed to be removed. The cost of the procedure could not have been further from my mind at this point, and faced with this life-changing possibility, I sat anxiously in the waiting room, thinking about the health of my wife and the possibility that I may not ever get to be called "Dad." Fortunately, after what seemed like an eternity, the doctor appeared in the waiting room to inform me of the surgical success. They were able to remove the cysts and save the ovaries, and I would be able to join my wife in the recovery room within the hour.

The remainder of the afternoon went just as planned. Within a few hours, we were discharged and on our way home. While Jenna, my wife, would spend the next few days in bed and a few additional weeks recovering from the operation, our return to daily life was imminent, and all was right with the world. Roughly a month following the surgery, I received the first of what would become numerous bills in the mail. There was the invoice from the anesthesiologist, and then from the surgical assistant. Another from the lab arrived, as well as some from other "ancillary" providers; then, finally, the hospital bill. The total charges would extend into the tens of thousands of dollars. Could this be right? Curious, I contacted the hospital and requested a detailed list of charges that were consolidated on the original invoice.

When I received the detailed listing, I was astounded. A sea of charges for things like pain medication, therapies, supplies, and personnel were all associated with various codes and acronyms; the listing might as well have been written in Greek for all the good it did me, and I felt I needed a quantum physics degree to try to decipher the various line items. The explanation of benefits I received from our insurance company would try to provide some clarity, outlining the billable charges, along with the network discounts. It listed those things *not* covered by our plan, along with portions of the procedure that were, and finally, the amount that we *may* owe. While, in the end, our "out-of-pocket" expense following the slew of discounts and contracted agreements was only a fraction of the total amount billed, I was amazed at the overall stated costs associated with what amounted to half a day's work.

This event took health care from being a job to being personal, and in the years that followed, our family found ourselves on the receiving end of the health care system many times; however, because of what I learned about the significance of actual medical billing (not just what I pay through insurance), I never let a bill simply come in and get paid. I would (and still do) always ask for a detailed bill, not just a summary. Just in the services my family would receive in the few years that followed, by diving into the bills, I would find thousands of dollars that were incorrectly invoiced—things like the lab that billed us for $800 following the birth of my son. Upon receiving the bill, I referenced it against my insurance company's EOB, only to find that the insurance company had already paid the lab. After I brought this to the lab's attention, the billing department of the lab stated that it was an accounting error and that the invoice had gone before it noted the receipt of insurance funds within its system. Another error occurred when I received two invoices for my portion of the deductible from the hospital in which I received spinal surgery in 2015. After hours on the phone with the billing department, disputing the charges (and getting nowhere), I finally took it upon myself to drive to the hospital, and within five minutes of sitting down with the billing specialist, the billing department removed the extra charges. These are just two examples of dozens of erroneous charges that, had I not been paying attention, I would have paid, thinking they were dollars I owed. And these don't even include the outrageous charges that I uncovered that were accurate (like the $8 tissue or the $8,000 I.V. bag), but we'll get into that in a later chapter.

For purposes of this discussion, I do not want to play up to any conspiracy theories out there or to give credence to the thought that billing errors just mean that hospitals are trying to get away with charging you more. On the whole, providers are not purposely fouling up your bill for the sake of wringing more money out of you or your insurer. Does that happen? Oh, absolutely. Just this past year, in 2018, the Department of Health and Human Services, along with the Department of Justice, prosecuted the largest ever health care fraud, charging over 600 defendants, with 165 of them being medical professionals, including 32 doctors. While intentional overbillings (or inaccurate billings) may occur most often, they are done so in error, not by intention. As stated in Hanlon's razor: "*Never attribute to malice that which is adequately explained by stupidity.*"[38] The average error is committed by individuals just like you and me, who are often overworked, underpaid, moving too fast, and who typed something wrong into the keyboard, which is not hard to do in health care, considering that the ICD-10 coding system has over 87,000 medical codes; it seems that, more often than not, the wrong code will get typed in. The issue here is that the system realizes that these errors occur, but it also realizes that most of us aren't paying attention. A practice that has been adopted recently during hospital and insurance company network negotiations is that of "auto adjudication" of claims. In short, this process allows a provider the ability to submit claims without being properly reviewed for errors (which, more often than not, leads to increased profits to the provider). Why would an insurance company agree to allow this? Remember that insurance companies are just finance companies now—the more they finance, the more they make. I remember a few years ago when someone on our team brought to my attention an invoice from a client for nearly $250,000. The procedure had been a knee scope—a service that typically runs somewhere between $15,000 and $30,000 at the most—so, of course, it caught our attention. After our team contacted the facility in which this service was rendered, we discovered that the $250,000 charge was actually a typographical error when the charges had been keyed in. The decimal point had been put in the wrong place, taking a $25,000 surgery to $250,000. Why didn't the insurance company catch this, you might ask? After an inquiry, it was uncovered that this specific procedure fell under its auto adjudication agreement with the provider, which meant that it was paid without appropriate review.

The moral of this story and the obvious solution here is that consumers *must* start looking at medical bills in closer detail. Never blindly trust the summary statement. But what about what I just said about there being no conspiracy? There isn't—just because the errors aren't being done maliciously doesn't mean they aren't there; roughly 80 percent of all medical bills contain billing errors.[39] I'm willing to bet you've received medical care more than once in your life, which means it's likely you've been billed incorrectly at some point. Being incorrectly billed doesn't necessarily mean the direct cost to you has gone up, but it does increase the chance that your insurance companies have simply been passing along those additional costs to you by way of increased insurance premiums. With claims of over $10,000, the chance of error has increased; according to Equifax, those bills often come with errors totaling more than $1,300.[40]

As a consumer, you should always request the line item of your doctor's bill; doctors are required, by law, to provide one to you. Some doctor's offices will try to dodge this requirement, but you need to buckle down and be patient and persistent. If, when you receive the bill, you have difficulty understanding the charges, call and speak to the billing department at the office and have them explain the charges to you. This is your health and your income—they are important. You owe it to yourself to get your money's worth. Some patients are worried that, by questioning their doctors, they may compromise their future health services. "*I have never seen that happen*," says Victoria Caras, founder of Aspen Medical Billing Advocates. "*Most of the time a doctor doesn't even know what the cost of their services are—they have outside billing agencies.*"[41] As I've said before, it's not the doctors running the industry anymore; it's the businesspeople.

Business practices can be devious; one, in particular, is called "balance billing" (sometimes referred to as "surprise billing"). Balance billing refers to a physician's ability to bill the patient for an outstanding balance after the insurance company submits its portion of the bill. More often than not, this results in a patient being "surprised" for a service they believed to be in-network and therefore covered by their insurance. This is not an uncommon practice, either; according to Kaiser Health News, 18 percent of people with coverage through a large employer who were admitted to a hospital in 2016 received at least one bill from an out-of-network provider.[42] In today's medical world, emergency rooms are heavily to blame for this practice; according to a health services research paper, 68 percent of inpatient involuntary contact with out-of-network physicians was related to the ER.[43] The rise in balance billing can be correlated to a lack of transparency in the ER space with patients. Seventy percent of patients were unaware that they had received out-of-network care, until they received a balance bill in the mail.[44]

Drew Calver, a Texas schoolteacher, suffered a severe heart attack in 2017 and was rushed to St. David's Medical Center. He was balance-billed $109,000 dollars for his four days in the hospital, even though his insurance was accepted at that facility; the medical center had covered only $56,000. "*I feel like I was exploited at the most vulnerable time of my life*," Calver said.[45] And he should feel that way; there is little in the way of consumer protection for someone like Calver, because his school district is self-funded, meaning it is a union or a group that pays claims out of its own funds and thus oftentimes forfeits any local- or state-based protections. These types of plans are regulated by a federal law called ERISA, the Employee Retirement Income Security Act of 1974, and neither ERISA or any other federal legislation prevents balance billing.

The simplest way to stop the practice of balance billing would be done through federal legislation that would apply to both state-regulated and self-funded plans, and that legislation would prohibit balance billing when someone visits an in-network facility but receives care from an out-of-network doctor. The wording of the legislation to be written would need to be broad enough to apply to all services relating to that care: imaging, lab testing, anesthesiology, and so forth, as well as facility fees and charges relating to the specific buildings where the care is administered. Additionally, the wording must be also be specific enough to not provide loop-holes for the industry to take advantage of; for example, to have imaging or other services conducted in a separate out-patient building next to the hospital, or some variant therein, in order to attempt avoiding the new legislation preventing balance-billing.

In the meantime, this struggle falls to the states. More than twenty states already have varying forms of consumer protection, ranging from mediation services to restrictions on balance billing in certain emergency situations. These are not limited to either conservative or liberal issues, either. In my home state of Texas, current proposals to limit balance billing have support from groups like the AARP and the Texas Hospital Association, as well as the left-leaning Center for Public Policy Priorities and the right-leaning Texas Conservative Coalition. "*It says something when you have two think tanks like CPPP and TCC on the same page on this*," replies Mia McCord, president of the TCC. And she's correct; as partisan as we've become in the United States, we should take note when our leaders find common ground. Republican Senator Kelly Hancock of suburban Fort Worth filed a bill in the Texas legislature, hoping to extend the modest protections that are provided to consumers to protect them from these larger companies; and State Representative Trey Martinez Fischer, a Democrat from San Antonio, filed a similar bill in the House.[46] Currently, the burden of resolving a claim rests on the consumer, and what hope does one individual have against the power of a multibillion dollar company? The average person can't compete with a system purposely built to limit their access to information, let alone take on the team of lawyers that exist to uphold the billing departments charges. Under the new Texas legislation, both sides of the payment dispute settle their issues through an existing balance-bill mediation program, currently handed through the TDI, the Texas Department of Insurance.

These programs are designed to apply in situations where patients don't have any choice about which facility they go to or about which physician is involved in their care. Health care companies may state this is a rarity, but when the program started in 2014, the department was asked to mediate 686 medical bills. During the 2018 fiscal year, it received 4,445 bills.[47] The program so far has saved Texas patients over $30 million, but this only helps when patients know these programs are available. Stacey Pogue, a senior policy analyst with the Center for Public Policy Priorities, says that patients often don't know these programs exist at all. "*The instructions for how to do it are on your medical bill and your explanation of benefits – the most indecipherable documents you are going to get,*"[48] Stacey says. Having these programs be available to the consumer at the state level is a great start, but clearly, we have a long way to go as we once again follow the money.

Because the money trail often ends, and without enough cash to cover the final cost, medical debt is one of the largest contributors to personal bankruptcy filings in the United States. In 2014, an estimated 40 percent of Americans racked up debt resulting from a medical issue.[49] "*Despite gains in coverage and access to care from the ACA, our findings suggest that it did not change the proportion of bankruptcies with medical causes,*"[50] says a study published in the *American Journal of Public Health*. During interviews conducted by the Kaiser Family Foundation on how medical debt has negatively affected their lives, patients provided responses such as the following: "*Have to take cold showers, can't fix plumbing. Other repairs have been patched as best as possible but not fixed.*" Another respondent stated, "*I am losing my house.*" And a common, but horrifying, comment: "*Charges for my insulin exceeded $1200 a month (3x my house payment). I had to reduce the amount of insulin I took based on what I could afford; my health was negatively impacted as a result.*"[51] Having to deal with medical issues is enough of a burden in and of itself, but the high costs associated with medical expenses are affecting patients' lives in serious and terrible ways. Of those queried, 70 percent said they cut back spending on food, clothing, or basic household items.

Another 41 percent took on an extra job or worked extra hours, and 26 percent had to take money out of retirement, college, or other long-term savings accounts. Even more alarming, 62 percent of patients had to rely on home remedies or over-the-counter drugs rather than seeing a doctor, and 43 percent did not fill a prescription for medicine they had been prescribed. It is this last statistic that may be the most concerning, as it leads us to understand that those 43 percent had already spent valuable money and time to see a doctor, but then could not afford to complete treatment because the medicine was too expensive. This is wrong, plain and simple. We must do better.

On the whole, Americans are not frivolously spending money on health care, at least not intentionally. Underhanded legal practices and loopholes in insurance contracts give greater protection to the hospitals and finance mechanisms than they do to the consumer. And this is where we need more oversight.

CHAPTER 9

Fee for Service

A lack of transparency may be the number one issue within our US health care system today—because a free market system doesn't work properly if the consumer doesn't have the information—but a very close second issue is how we compensate providers for services rendered. In the United States, health care is delivered on what is called a "fee-for-service" model. In short, this means we pay for everything we get along the way versus paying for the end result. Every test, every lab, every doctor, every nurse, every practitioner, and even every tissue is a different unbundled billable service within our system. Many within the medical industry will claim that there is no way to sustain the system while removing this structure; at the very least, we should realign the incentives. Today, the delivery system is incentivized to run more tests, to perform more procedures, and even to have patients remain in a hospital rather than being discharged. The fee-for-service model ensures this and was only fueled by what may have been the single worst provision within the Affordable Care Act.

As part of the ACA, insurance companies could no longer implement what were known as "lifetime maximums" on the amount they would pay out on claims for any individual person (typically the maximums were between $1 million and $5 million, on average). Again, while those that drafted the legislation were including this portion of the law with the best of intentions, it led to the worst of outcomes. In the twenty years I've been involved in the health care industry and with all of the claims I've reviewed over those years and in all the time leading up to the ACA, rarely did I see a claim exceed more than $1 million, and I never saw anything near a payout of $5 million. Post-ACA, a bill of $1 million is not uncommon, and an amount over $5 million is not unlikely. By including this provision, lawmakers gave hospital systems a blank check with which to run up the tab. You might be thinking, *But if the health insurers are on the hook for that, why wouldn't they be averse to these massive claims?* They may be fronting the money, but rest assured they're collecting it in insurance premiums. Let's take a frustrating look at the average stock prices of insurance companies in the time since the passage of the Affordable Care Act. The first number represents their average stock prices in early 2010, pre-ACA, and the second number represents their average stock prices at the beginning of 2019.

United Healthcare: $32.18 to $262.12[52]
Anthem (BCBS): $63.94 to $311.58[53]
Cigna Corporation: $33.36 to $217.65[54]

President Obama said it best himself, with such high hopes before the ACA was passed, during a press conference on July 22, 2009: "*I want to talk to you a bit about the progress we are making on health-insurance reform and how it fits into our broader economic strategy.*"[55]

Did you catch that? The ACA was never about health care reform; it was about health insurance reform, and on the basis of the profits of these insurers, they were certainly reformed. By focusing only on one aspect of the industry as a whole and by not taking cost containment into consideration, the Affordable Care Act, as it was written, was doomed to fail and has led to serious consequences.

In the winter of 2018, my daughter contracted a very serious stomach flu. After we consulted with her pediatrician, given that she was only three years old, it was recommended that we take her to our local children's hospital so that she could have an IV administered. She was in the hospital for fewer than twenty-four hours and received a treatment consisting of two IV-fluid bags for dehydration, along with some observation by nurses and occasional conversations with a few doctors. Total bill: $16,000. Did the two IV bags cost $8,000 apiece? No, of course not, but the hospital had billed us, using the fee-for-service model, or what's also referred to as an unbundled rate. We weren't being billed for just what was used; we were billed on the basis of what was available to be used. Picture a hospital room: all the tubing, every latex glove that a nurse could put on, the soap at each sink that's available for washing hands, and the box of tissues, if needed. For every single item there was a charge. This means that while we were in the hospital for twenty-two hours, because those hours ran into a second day (after midnight), the hospital had the right per its insurance network contract agreement to bill for three boxes of latex gloves (small, medium, and large) for two days. If you're wondering, *No, there weren't that many pairs of gloves used*, and when you consider that the actual cost of a box of latex gloves is approximately $5.00 but that is often billed by hospitals as much as $175 per box, you can see how easy it is for bills from a hospital can be outrageous and, dare I say, egregious. During our stay, in addition to products our daughter used (two IV bags and a few latex gloves), the hospital had the right to bill for every nurse that came in and for every doctor who reviewed a chart.

While we may never see a system completely removed from fee-for-service, there are various alternative payment methods (APMs) that could alleviate our current platform. One solution would be to switch to a bundled-payer system. In this scenario, if a patient presents with a heart condition, the hospital charges a flat rate for that heart condition, not a rate for how many cardiologists it gathered in the room to give their opinion. Regardless of how many tests, blood workups, and medications are prescribed, all charges would fall under the one episode of care. Hospitals are vehemently opposed to this change in payer care for obvious monetary reasons. Currently, the burden of debt falls onto the patient, regardless of the amount of treatment or how many tests are run to determine the condition. When patients are admitted to the hospital, included in the small novel of paperwork the patients are expected to read and sign is a promissory note to pay. Even though they didn't know they were about to buy a Toyota Camry or, in some cases, a Lamborghini, the patients swear to uphold their financial end of the deal. In essence, they are writing a blank check to the hospital saying, "Fix me," and even if they are unable to do so, the patients will be billed for all the hospital's efforts.

Many of us still picture the Norman Rockwell version of our doctor, our friend in a white lab coat. We trust our doctors implicitly, even if we've never met them before, and when we are in a hospital, doctors seem to carry even more gravity. So when patients are told that they need more tests or that they are going to be sent upstairs, they have this absolute faith that since doctors are part of the health care system, they are navigating the complexities on behalf of the patients and in their best interests. As has been stated and will be stated again, the medical industry is a business, and the doctors within it make their money on tests and treatments. Since ordering extra tests doesn't harm the patient and since most of the tests will end up being covered by insurance anyway, it's easy to justify inflating the costs.[56] Let me be clear: most doctors genuinely want nothing more than to help their patients, and extra tests do indeed rule things out, even if they're confident in the results. But remember this, too: it's not the doctors running the health care system; it's the businesspeople in suits who are looking at P&L.[57] Doctors often have quotas,[58] which is as large of a conflict of interest as can be found in any other industry. The person responsible for a patient's care should never have ulterior motives for assigning one version of treatment or another.

In a bundled-payment model, the patient pays the providers involved by using a set price for the episode of care. The price associated with that care is set on the basis of historical costs, taking into account the average number of tests it takes to establish the condition. Those costs can inflate regularly, on the basis of the overall cost of delivering the goods sold (just as they would in any other industry). If the providers exceed the prearranged reimbursement for a specific episode, they should be the ones to bear the financial responsibility for overages, preventing balance billing (surprise billing) for the patient. This method would encourage standardized, cost-effective care decisions and pairs well with the released prices of the hospital charge masters that happened recently.[59] There are challenges when this method of payment is used for patients who have several comorbidities, some of which are high risk, as this can introduce expenses that would be unfairly placed on the hospital during that "episode of care." There would need to be reasonable allowance for multiple claims to be filed against an episode of care in the instance of severe comorbidities that affected the patient's stay at the hospital. Remember: the hallmark of a good compromise is that no one walks away happy—if we suggest improvements to paying the hospitals, they have to be fair and balanced, not just lowering the costs for the patients.

A bundled-payment option is not without its possible implications. It would be possible that hospitals will "encourage" their doctors to go with the most cost-effective treatments or to run as few tests as needed, which is why transparency is so necessary. Have you been to a restaurant in any metropolitan area lately? Likely upon entering the establishment, you saw, in plain sight, a large placard with the letter A. The placard shows how the health department has reviewed the restaurant and the quality in which its health standards are ranked. If you see a placard with a B or a C in the window, you'll likely go somewhere else for your meal. If we are so concerned that we may eat food that hasn't been properly handled that we require restauranteurs (who are required to have no training or degree to open a restaurant, I might add) to post their health department ratings, shouldn't we do the same for hospitals and doctors' offices? This would likely prevent health care providers or facilities from shortchanging their patients by way of inadequate care or diagnosis. In a free market, to keep a system accountable, the consumer *must* have the information. The consumer now has decision-making power, and the government cannot set prices. Competition is allowed to thrive, and the best health care at the most effective price wins. The patient must be able to view the pricing structures within the health care system, a listing of the procedures that are available, and their associated costs. This method will ensure accountability and a higher level of quality outcomes. The end result would be that providers aren't just ordering whatever helps their bottom line; rather, the providers are doing what is most appropriate for their patients.

A great method of removing misaligned incentives and keeping the physician thinking solely about the patient is utilized by the Cleveland Clinic in Ohio. The beauty of its methodology lies in the simplicity of the solution: pay doctors a healthy salary, and allow no incentivizing of the medical staff. Within the walls of a hospital, the number of industry-related sales reps is endless. We often think about the pharmaceutical reps, but there are also salespeople for all types of medical equipment, like MRI machines and ventilators; reps selling the types of metals used in knee replacements; even reps for the latex gloves utilized by the hospital's medical staff. These salespeople will use multiple tactics to get their products to be the ones preferred by providers within the facility. While various sales tactics and incentives may be deployed at hospitals throughout the country, they are not deployed at the Cleveland Clinic. There are pharmacy reps offering free trips to exotic locales to see that latest brand of pain killer or kickbacks or reward structures for certain amounts of pills prescribed. No misaligned (financial) influences from medical equipment reps or from those selling any products of any kind. The amazingly simple act of removing the incentives for the doctors means that they will pick which pills to prescribe, what surgeries to perform, and what tests to be undertaken on the basis of the best outcome for the patient at the best price for the hospital system.

As we have discussed, removing the incentives is a multifunctional and massively effective solution. By realigning goals and objectives between doctors and patients, health care develops into a more impactful and personal relationship. It is no longer dependent on how many patients are seen, how many tests and procedures ordered, or the overall margin generated to the bottom line. By doing the right things, however, as is proved by the Cleveland Clinic (which is often revered as the most effective heart hospital in the nation—perhaps the world), profits and the bottom line are still positive, along with patient outcomes and experience. At the Cleveland Clinic, doctors are hired on yearly contracts, and their metrics for success are tied to fewer readmissions, infection rates, length of recovery, and medical errors. Additionally, doctors are reviewed on clinical outcomes and research.[60] This is assisted by the strategies that more minds are better than one and that patients are not seen by only one attending physician. Teams support each other, and while it's true that one doctor per patient is faster, it isn't necessarily better. New approaches like these are the start towards value-based care, which, in turn, can help lead us to outcome-based care.

CHAPTER 10

There's a Pill for That

The rising costs of prescription drugs are one of the most tangible challenges with which nearly every American can identify. Within the United States in 2017, 85.1 percent[61] of adults saw a health care professional, and 93.6 percent of children did so as well.[62] As a result of those visits, over 4.45 billion prescriptions were issued.[63] Think about that number for a moment. With a total population of approximately 327 million in the United States, given the number of scripts, that would mean an average of thirteen prescriptions per person. Of the total expenditure on health care, 17.9 percent[64] of that spending is on pharmaceutical drugs, or $339 billion. Americans average more than $1,000 per person per year on pills.

Now that's some big business. Out of every $6.00, $1.00 is spent on health care, with $1.00 of every $6.00 of those being spent on prescription drugs. Like all things in the tangle that is the health care industry, there is no single problem or a single conspirator to blame when it comes to the ever-rising costs of prescription drugs.

It is a knot of problems and pricing tangling unto itself like the Gordian knot. Unlike that legendary knot, we cannot simply slice our way to a solution. We must follow the larger strands to where they lead and identify solutions, one at a time.

Happiness Is Just a Pill Away

Let's begin with how drugs are marketed within the United States. For as long as people have existed, someone has been peddling a solution to health-related problems. Early on within the United States, traveling salesmen marketed a cure for creaky joints, powders to keep the face young and beautiful, and even the secret to eternal life (or so they claimed). Remember that Coca-Cola® was originally sold in 1885 for its "medicinal" ingredients: kola nuts and cocaine.[65] To help combat this Wild West of misinformation and snake oil, the Food and Drug administration (FDA) was founded in 1906 to slowly begin regulating serious abuses in the consumer-product marketplace.[66] It wouldn't happen until 1951 that drugs became properly classified into a "prescription" drug or a "nonprescription" drug, as there had been no process before 1951. In the decades that followed World War II, with new drugs and treatments being developed at breakneck speed, the need to have properly trained and engaged physicians administer access of possibly harmful (yet impactful) drugs became law. Drug manufacturers would be required to submit information regarding their latest and greatest developments to doctors and pharmacists, who, in turn, would make recommendations to their patients on the basis of their specific medical needs.

That process all changed when, in May of 1983, the first television ad for a prescription drug aired (a pain-relief medication called Rufen), and direct-to-consumer advertising (DTA) was born. The FDA tried to stop this DTA advertising scheme, but with the help of PhRMA and the marketing power that the medical lobbying industry wielded, they were unsuccessful. That marketing strategy continues today, with nearly $30 billion spent each year on drug marketing and advertising.[67] No longer do the average consumers learn of the merits of a particular drug from their doctor; instead, the marketing system allows for prescription drug manufacturers to address them directly through television, print, and radio ads. In a system that restricts the consumers from directly purchasing these goods without the consent and authorization from their physicians, why would it be necessary to speak directly to those who can't self-prescribe? Why take on the huge expense? Because these ads feed on the consumers' fears and desires. Picture the last advertisement you saw for a particular drug where you likely saw something akin to soft sunsets and handsome actors engaging in activities both fun and pain-free. We all aspire to be as carefree as those depicted in the pharmaceutical commercials, and for those possibly dealing with painful or even life-threatening diseases, wouldn't it be great to be as happy and symptom-free as those actors they see in the ads? More than just happy: combine that emotion with the fear of not pursuing all options available in their treatments of difficult illnesses, and the consumers are eager to do just about anything to heal, including questioning whether their doctors know if a promoted treatment is available.

As a capitalist, I'm not opposed to any businesses promoting their products, but in the United States, the patient is too heavily influenced by limited information. The patient should be informed, but not through a catchy jingle and a TV model dancing through an open field. As was the case early on, the physician should be the primary avenue of information regarding the merits of a drug, not a thirty-second spot between *American Idol* auditions.

The solution to our first issue is simple but difficult: the government needs to help those who aren't in a position to always consider all of the facts. This can be accomplished with more oversight and more transparency in medical advertising. Advertising is essential in disseminating information, but to utilize it as a source of persuasion is a massive misuse of the microphone (or television screen, for that matter). Since we are not likely to go the route of almost every other nation, outlawing the advertising of drugs, we should focus on what could be accomplished. In the same way that HHS has recently mandated that hospital charge masters be made public, so too a similar policy should be applied to medical advertising in all of its forms. At the time of the publishing of this book, the Trump Administration, under the leadership of HHS Secretary Alex Azar, has taken the initial steps to do this very thing. For prescriptions, however, this is not as straightforward as giving consumers their list price in the commercial, which HHS has stated it wants to pursue. These drugs pass through many hands in their creation—from research and development, to production, to purchase by the wholesaler (the PBMs), to sales to the pharmacy themselves; they are price-gouged numerous times on their journey to the end user. Therefore, the prices that must be made public are what they are at the start of their journey—the price of the pill sold to the PBM. This informs the public when a prescription that began at $10 per pill ends with a $200 pill. Since further mandates would be needed to show the pricing at every step of the way, this would be a solid first step. We will cover PBMs a little further ahead.

The Price of the Potion

Another major contributor to the rising cost of health care is how expensive it is to actually manufacture new drugs. At first blush, that sounds like a cop-out. When you look at large companies like Johnson & Johnson, who spent $17.5 billion on marketing but only $8.2 billion on R&D, all the while reporting $13.8 billion in profit,[68] it can be hard to feel any sympathy on the side of the pharmaceutical companies, and I'm certainly not asking you to. But we get to look at it through the lens of the past. For many drug companies, it takes, on average, twelve years and $2.6 billion to bring a successful new drug to market.[69] Additionally, only 10 percent of all Phase I products receive FDA approval, so the creation of a successful money-making drug is far from a sure thing. We want pharmaceutical companies to cure diseases. We want them to come up with new drugs. We want them to continue to advance medicine. In a world where we had measles, mumps, rubella, and polio, we needed the pharmaceutical companies. And while we need to ensure accuracy in diligence in the development of new medicines, we also need to loosen the restraints of the federal government and how they require pharmaceutical companies to bring a drug to market. If we are able to combine the transparency of pricing with the HHS mandates, then assisting the pharmaceutical companies in developing drugs at lower prices benefits us all, as it allows new companies to compete (where financially they may not have been able to) and reduces the overhead of development, resulting in lower prices for the drugs themselves.

One of the easiest solutions in shortening the time from study to market is to soften the language that allows research from foreign countries to be used in FDA approval. The FDA does allow foreign research, but currently, the 1983 version of legislation in effect is unnecessarily strict in its language usage regarding foreign clinical research. In October of 2000, the World Medical Association revised the declaration, but the FDA chose not to incorporate those revisions into its regulations.[70] This was a curious choice; the WMA is a group of physicians over 10 million strong, led by countries which include the United States, Germany, Japan,

Sweden, and Israel.[71] These are trusted allies and are well-proven in the safety of their scientific research and whose recommendations should be accepted in our government's regulations. So, in effect, the United States does not allow foreign research to prove efficacy or safety, and therefore, the research must be duplicated by American companies to prove the same effects. Clinical research takes the better part of a decade[72]; and with the average cost to the manufacturer being $712,000 per day,[73] any shortening of time bringing that new drug to market would pay dividends in the creation of new drugs, ideally resulting in lower prices for consumers.

Of course, there must be restrictions in the loosening of any FDA regulations. A major concern of physicians is that politicians would go too far in trying to please drug manufacturers, which is a distinct possibility, given the power of the lobbying force in that industry. We must mandate that any loosening of regulations does not hamper the FDA's ability to rigorously evaluate the safety and the effectiveness of new drugs and that drug manufacturers must still demonstrate efficacy, alongside safety, as a condition for market entry. There should be balance in all things; if we can produce medicines faster and cheaper, that's wonderful, but we must be sure they work and are safe for consumers.

The Patient Problem

When new drug formulas are invented, before all of the testing, research, and trials, they are patented with the US Patent and Trademark Office, at which point the clock begins. Starting immediately, those drug manufacturers will have twenty years of protection, but before they can sell their product included in that time frame, they must also perform all refinement, study, preclinical, in vitro, and in vivo research to prepare for the FDA drug review and approval, a process that, in and of itself, is no quick feat. With luck, those billions were well-spent, and a new drug is ready to generate profit for its creator. But while exclusivity was supposed to be an incentive for the generation of new and societally beneficial products, it has turned into a weapon wielded by the pharmaceutical companies for ever-expanding pursuits of higher profits. Let me be clear: I'm not trying to prohibit an organization from making a profit—and a fair profit, at that. Nor am I suggesting that the FDA or any department of the federal government restrict the rights of a drug manufacturer, but what I am suggesting is that Uncle Sam needs to stop the practice of long-term competition protection.

It's estimated that once a generic drug hits the market after a patent expiration, brand name sales drop by 80 percent and that, over time, the price of the original brand name drug lowers by nearly 60 percent.[74] This is great news to the consumer, who now has access to more options and is paying lower prices. This is, however, not-so-welcome news to the shareholders of the original manufacturer and to those pharmaceutical companies that have a fiduciary responsibility to provide the most profit as possible, which leads many to engage in a number of questionable practices that satisfy the letter of the law but blatantly violate the spirit of it.

When Humira was originally released by drug manufacturer Abbot Laboratories (now AbbVie) in 2002, it was intended to treat patients suffering from rheumatoid arthritis. Today, it is marketed to treat conditions from ankylosing spondylitis (spine inflammation) to ulcerative colitis, plaque psoriasis, idradenitis suppurativa (skin disease), Crohn's disease, and ingrown toenails (okay, I made the last one up, but I'm sure Abbvie is working on it). Today, as a result of both original and new patents being issued, AbbVie holds over 130 patents for Humira, and given its numerous extensions, a generic or biosimilar version of the drug isn't likely to come to market anytime soon. In fact, several of the patents on Humira (over 100 of them) are currently scheduled through 2034, meaning that AbbVie will have had at least thirty-two years of market exclusivity before the patent is available for an American generic. By routinely finding new uses for the drug, many of which seem conveniently discovered shortly before the patent is set to run out, AbbVie is able to apply for extensions that cover the drug as a whole. As a consequence, there is no generic alternative for Humira with which to treat rheumatoid arthritis (whose patent expired) because of the patent extension by Abbvie for Humira to treat Crohn's disease. This is a clear gaming of the system at the expense of the patient and consumer. The biosimilars that have been created in Europe for a generic version of Humira (by Amgen and Novartis) are currently available overseas at less than $10,000 annually (more than 80 percent less than the average cost of Humira in the United States) because the European Union has far less patience than the United States when it comes to medical lobbying. In the meantime, Americans will continue having to pay the more than $50,000 average annual cost of Humira, until its patents run out here in the United States.[75] Again, there currently exists a functioning, manufactured generic in Europe, but it isn't allowed here because of patent extension. A possible solution for extreme prescription costs is to allow certain foreign markets to sell approved drugs in the United States. As a capitalist, I am all for free trade, and while it exists in many aspects of our economy, the drug industry, along with all of its players, has successfully prevented the "free trade" of prescriptions here in the United States.

Mash-Up

Another trend in prescription-drug development and marketing is what many refer to as the development of "stupid drugs." A drug manufacturer will take two previously released drugs (sometimes over-the-counter medications), combine them into a single pill, file a patent, and then market the new drug as innovative treatment. Let's take, for example, Vimovo, which is typically used to treat patients with early signs of rheumatoid arthritis. Often, patients dealing with chronic pain and inflammation will take a nonsteroidal anti-inflammatory medication called naproxen (sold as "over the counter" under the brand name Aleve). One side effect of naproxen is that it can sometimes cause stomach pain and even ulcers. As such, many times patents will take esomeprazole magnesium (sold "over the counter" under the name brand Nexium) to alleviate this pain and prevent the possibility of stomach ulcers. As mentioned above, both Aleve and Nexium can be purchased over the counter at any local drug store and will cost approximately $40. Vimovo, which is manufactured by Horizon Pharma, Inc. and has some patent protections though 2031, combines naproxen and esomeprazole magnesium into one pill rather than two and costs, on average, more than $2,500 for one month's supply. While I'm sure that the convenience of taking one drug instead of two might appeal to many patients, doing so at an increased price of 6,300 percent would likely or should likely prevent most patients from pursuing this course of action. Many physicians prescribe Vimovo to their patients today, because, to say it simply, the drug works—as it should, given that it's two previously proven drugs that have been on the market for years. Unfortunately, many doctors don't recognize that there may be a lower-cost option for their patients. This is often because they themselves don't know the extent of the cost of a drug like Vimovo. I don't meant to pick on this drug only; today, there are dozens of drugs on the market that have received patents and are being prescribed to patients who could instead take two generic or over-the-counter drugs rather than combining them into a single pill.

Herein lies the continued challenge of information because of a lack of transparency. If patients understood what has just been described, I would imagine that the vast majority of consumers would choose to take two pills instead of one and save themselves hundreds (possibly thousands) of dollars in the process. But unfortunately, as we talked about previously, the consumers aren't inundated with that kind of information in marketing. The doctors are not telling them, and the pharmaceutical companies certainly aren't, either. The patent office writes another short-term monopoly for a company, and the costs stay high. Taking two existing drugs and combining them into one should not be eligible for patent protection, and if it is, it should be eligible for patent protection for a much shorter period of time than what is standard.

The Compromise

There are several other strategies that exist within the patent-extension schemes, but what it boils down to is simple: the longer a company holds the patent, the longer generics are not able to be introduced; thus the higher cost (and profit) of drugs is maintained. This discourages competition, and in a free market society, competition is required to create a fair market. The solution would be to reduce these patent extensions or to place a cap on how many patents can be introduced, regardless of future changes. The Humira example of the never-ending patent is a clear indicator that the system needs change. Quid pro quo for consumers and companies both, the driving argument from manufacturers has been that, because of the length of time needed to generate new medicine, drug-patent extensions have been necessary to generate a meaningful profit. If we are able to reduce the cost of producing new drugs, via FDA deregulation, then the argument that patent extensions must be granted to generate a profit is severely undercut.

Pharmacy Benefit Managers

Quite possibly the most influential reason why prescription drugs are such a challenge within the United States lies in how the pricing is set and the drug distributed. It has long been thought that drugs are manufactured, then sold directly to the retail pharmacy by the pharmaceutical company. In turn, the insurance company, which ultimately pays for the drugs (less a patient's copay or coinsurance), negotiates what it will pay to the pharmaceutical company for the drug in question. While in the end, this process may be deemed as somewhat accurate, there are more layers to the prescription-drug supply chain, which yield significant profits for *all* parties involved—pay attention, and you'll learn about the real "collusion" going on in America today.

In the early days of the modern health care system, many insurance plans didn't cover prescription drugs, because only a few generations ago, the variety of prescription drugs was limited, and the costs weren't all that much. By the 1960s, however, more advancements in medicine meant more prescription drugs, more manufacturers developing those drugs, and more consumers utilizing prescription drugs as a regular part of their care. As a result, insurance companies began covering the cost of prescriptions, and, because of the administrative challenges of claims, formularies, and price negotiations, a new division of the health care industry was established, the pharmacy benefit manager. These "PBMs," as they became known, would essentially be the go-betweens, or middlemen, negotiating between the drug manufacturers and the insurance companies. As compensation, the PBMs would charge fees on the basis of the number of claims processed. By the

1980s, the PBMs were the primary intermediaries in the drug-distribution model.[76]

While the process has seen little adjustment over the past fifty years, the ways in which PBMs are compensated for their work have changed immensely (as have the profits). Today, PBMs generate revenue in one of three ways:

1. Fees—just as in their early years, PBMs often still charge fees on the basis of the number of prescriptions they process and the drugs they negotiate for distribution.
2. Rebates—we'll refer to these as "spiff" bonuses paid to the PBMs based on the volume of drugs distributed. The rebates are often referred to as discounts, and the PBMs historically have kept the rebates as additional profits in addition to their fees.
3. Spread—this is the profit generated from the variance between what the PBM negotiates on the price of the drug from the manufacturer and the price for which it then sells it to the pharmacy—the spread.

The original purpose of PBMs was to reduce cost by streamlining administration and distribution, along with improving access to appropriate medications. Today, many believe PBMs have become more the culprits in the rising cost of prescription drugs and less the advocates. From 1987 to 2014, the economy grew 126 percent, and consumer spending grew 169 percent; however, during that same time, spending increased by 1,010 percent.[77] The actual dollar amount spent on prescriptions in the United States has risen from $26.8 billion in 1987 to nearly $500 billion today. PBMs will point to things like the development of high-cost specialty drugs and the overall increased drug prices as the reason behind these numbers, but while that may be partially true, PBMs have benefited from all of these as well.

The primary purpose of PBMs has shifted from that of driving costs down to that of returning the most profits. Look behind the curtain, and you will find that PBMs are no longer independent organizations but part of the finance mechanism of health care—health insurance. Nearly all major health insurers today own their PBMs, thus not only financing the premiums that pay for the prescription drugs on behalf of their customers but also profiting from them as well—talk about a conflict of interest. Nearly 75 percent of all drugs distributed in the United States today are done so by one of three PBMs, all of which are either owned by (or own) a health insurance company (Express Scripts and Cigna, Optum and United Healthcare, and CVS and Aetna). To bring this full circle, the PBM negotiates the price of the drug with the manufacturer. PBMs set the formularies, which direct the patients into which drugs they have access to and what prices through their insurance companies. PBMs generate profits by fees they charge to distribute the drugs, the spread based on the variance between the price by which they purchase the drugs and the price by which they sell the drugs. Finally, the PBMs generate profits by the rebates on the basis of how many particular drugs are sold. All this is financed by the consumer by way of insurance premiums, yet the insurance companies are parts of the PBMs—collusion, anyone?

The United States government must step in here and either force open transparency in how the system operates or break up the monopolistic way by which health care is distributed. There are some good PBMs in the United States that still hold true to their original intent of driving down costs and increasing access for consumers, but those PBMs hold very little market share and even less influence over the pharmaceutical industry. By allowing PBMs to be part of the insurance system, the prices of drugs remains inflated, consumers are less served, but profits remain high. It is a direct conflict of interest.

Hostile Negotiations

While to some, the idea of Uncle Sam stepping in to change how the current so called free enterprise of health care and, more specifically, how the distribution of prescription drugs operates is off-putting, many conservatives believe that there should be no government intervention at all. And while we may agree to disagree on that, one thing we may be able to agree on, especially if we apply the basics of capitalism, is that any enterprise purchasing any goods should have the ability to negotiate.

The federal government, via Medicare and Medicaid, is the single largest purchaser of pharmaceuticals in the country, estimated to be nearly 30 percent of the nation's spending on prescription drugs.[78] Despite that massive buying power, the government is forbidden by law against negotiating prices. What?

First, we need to speak about the power of the lobbying industry, known as PhRMA, the Pharmaceutical Research and Manufacturers of America. As part of the overall health care lobby, which is larger than oil and gas, tobacco, and defense lobbies combined,[79] PhRMA, along with its co-lobbying on behalf of health care groups, has had significant influence in this issue, particularly. Before we get into the specifics of how lobbying has influenced how the government procures drugs, it's important to note that more than 60 percent of the lobbyists are what are known as "revolvers," that is, lobbyists who previously served in Congress or who worked as congressional aides or in other government jobs. This naturally raises suspicion that lawmakers and regulators will go easy on the industry to not jeopardize their chances of lucrative jobs after leaving office or not affecting future donations to their campaigns. In 2016, there were 894 healthcare lobbyists hired to influence the 535 members of Congress. That's almost two lobbyists per congressman, full time, but I digress.

Back to prescriptions and how Uncle Sam buys them: in 2003, Congress approved a landmark program to help senior citizens buy prescription drugs. Rather than senior citizens' directly purchasing drugs within the Medicare system, it would be up to the insurance companies who would be delivering the subsidized new coverage, known as Medicare Part D (it's important here to note who owns the PBMs, which profit from the distribution of drugs).

This leads us to perhaps the most notorious example of lobbying corruption in the history of health care. Louisiana Congressman Billy Tauzin, who, as the chairman of the House Energy and Commerce Committee, helped write Medicare Part D legislation, known as the Medicare Modernization Act of 2003.[80] While serving as the committee chair, legislation was added to the MMA that denied the government the ability to negotiate prescription drug prices. A few years later, in January of 2005, immediately after retiring from Congress, Mr. Tauzin was hired as the president of PhRMA, where he remained at that top job until 2010, during which time he was paid a salary of $2 million a year.[81]

And there you have it.

The House Committee on Energy and Commerce was originally responsible for preventing the ability of the US government to directly negotiate the prices of drugs it purchases. To overturn this and write new legislation, the same committee would be tapped once again. The current chairman of the HCEC, Frank Pallone of New Jersey, has taken a total of $5,921,471 from the health care industries over the course of his political career.[82] According to the US Census Bureau, the lifetime income of the average American is $1.4 million.[83] In plain terms, the chairman has been given what could be considered four lifetimes of income in campaign contributions from the health care lobby, and he's not alone. Republican Fred Upton of Michigan has taken $3,339,123, and Democrat

Scott Peters of California has taken $1,062,224. Of the fifty-five members currently serving on the HCEC[84] (including members of both parties), all have received contributions from the health care lobby. In short, both sides of the political spectrum have taken tens of millions of dollars in contributions.[85]

According to a KFF poll, 93 percent of Democrats and 74 percent of Republicans favor letting the government negotiate Part D prices.[86] When the VA and IHA (Indian Health Service) negotiate prescription prices, they routinely acquire lower-priced medication. The numbers for how much savings would be generated by negotiations vary, but the Congressional Budgetary Office estimates the savings would average $11 billion per year[87] at the outset, with higher savings if the Secretary of HHS was granted authority to remove certain drugs from coverage.[88] So public opinion wants this, and politicians campaign on it, but nothing has changed. I wonder why?

CHAPTER 11

Health Insurance—The Tie That Binds

As was stated early on in this book, health insurance is *not* health care. They are two very different things, but, in the United States, the marketers of the status quo want the American public to think about them synonymously. One is the delivery of care, and the other is the financing of it. While the initial structure of health insurance dating back to its earliest days was to provide protection, today it's simply become the credit card and access point by which the public enters into the delivery system. Nearly 90 percent of Americans access the health care system through some form of insurance, whether that is private insurance, employer-sponsored insurance, or a government-run program. Between 2007 and 2017, health insurance premiums increased by 55 percent, while the overall inflation rate in the United States rose just over 18 percent. That's a more than 300 percent variance between the two. Given this information, there must be more going on behind the scenes, right? Yes—yes, there is, and we are falling right into the trap. If you want to really understand why health insurance premiums are increasing to the tune of three times the rate of everything else, look no further than the health care industry. Health insurance companies are the primary financier of the health care system. In other words and more specifically, Blue Cross Blue Shield, Aetna, Cigna and United Healthcare (to name a few) are really just the Visa and MasterCard of hospitals, doctors, and pharmaceuticals. Think about it: who pays cash for much of anything anymore? Whether we are buying groceries, a new television, or even movie tickets, instead of paying cash, we throw down our debit card or credit card (got to get those points, right?). In the same way, when we go into a doctor's office, the hospital, or local pharmacy, what's the first thing we reach for? That insurance ID card. Yep, feels kind of the same, right? But what makes all other transactions different than health care transactions is that we know the price of what we are paying for when it comes to every other thing we buy, but not when it comes to health care. When it comes to health care–related transactions, we think of the copay or the deductible, not the price, and, as a result, we fall right into the hands of both the health care system and the health insurance industry, which for decades approached each other more as rivals but which now seem to be collaborators.

In a post–Affordable Care Act world, the insurance market has seen massive consolidation, with many parts of the country having only one primary option within the private market. In its early years, health insurance policies were known as indemnity plans, offering participants financial protection against catastrophic occurrences. Throughout the years, policies evolved to cover more routine medical needs, like standard doctors' visits and prescription drugs. In an effort to drive new business, insurance companies formed networks, which gave their customers value, as doctors and hospitals would discount their services within each specific carrier's network. In exchange for their discounted services, the insurance companies would steer new patients to the provider. While this platform was sustainable for many years, as a result of insurance company consolidation, today many providers are in-network, with each of the available insurance networks rendering the discounts to be ineffective in actually driving down costs. Sure, many insurance companies will still tout their networks' value on the basis of the discounts, but as I often say, discounts don't matter; prices do. Hospital systems and insurance companies have found ways around the messaging of insurance discounts, often yielding the same amount of revenue, regardless of the network used, to the provider by way of how certain procedures are billed and bundled or unbundled. Today, networks are so similar in their outputs of value that they yield no unique benefit from one to another. Many Americans even find they receive better pricing on services by simply paying cash, in lieu of utilizing insurance.

While the Affordable Care Act's primary objective was to reform the US health insurance system, it empowered it instead and finalized its transformation into a true finance mechanism. As a result, while its intent was to reign in big insurance, the ACA actually propelled health insurance companies to never-before-seen profit levels, many of which have seen over 200 percent increases in their stock performance. While I do not believe we should eliminate insurance companies, and while I do not believe they should be nonprofit, we must reform the way in which they operate. Today, more than ever before, and in large part, because of the way the ACA was drafted, health insurance companies are aligned with the delivery system rather than its adversary. As I have stated before, one continues to be the commodity, and the other has become the credit card.

We are in desperate need of health insurance reform in the United States. We need to eliminate insurance networks and the nontransparent way in which contracts are negotiated between insurers and providers. Health insurance should return to its original intent, to protect the consumer from loss, rather than what it does today, which is financing the consumer's consumption. By eliminating insurance networks, we shine a light on the true pricing in the health care system, and consumers will make choices on the basis of the amount of coverage provided, not on the basis of some opaque discount hidden in a network negotiation. Eliminating insurance networks would also eliminate surprise billing and "out-of-network" charges. The price would be the price, and the insurance either would or would not cover the service. No more guessing.

The Affordable Care Act provided the platform, but it approached the market all wrong. It must be repealed and replaced or, at the very least, rebuilt from the ground up. We must maintain provisions like the protection for preexisting conditions and access to preventative care; however, we must realign the incentives and still offer the American public choices instead of mandates.

The Government Option

Contrary to the rhetoric, the United States does indeed have a "public option" today. As a matter of fact, nearly half of the population is already enrolled in this platform—it simply has a barrier to entry. Both Medicare and Medicaid are funded and managed by Uncle Sam, and, according the US Census Bureau, in 2017, roughly 130 million Americans were enrolled in one of the two government programs. Medicare is available to persons of a certain age or disability, and Medicaid is available to those of a certain income level. Some (specifically those on the left) believe that we should move to a Medicare For All platform. Senator Bernie

Sanders, the self-described democratic socialist from Vermont, has long promoted the idea of universal health care promoting a "single-payer" platform similar to what may be found in more socialized systems like those in Canada and throughout Europe. Here's the challenge: "Medicare For All," as proponents like to call it, isn't Medicare at all. In its current state, Medicare is divided into multiple parts (A, B, C, D), each offering various levels of coverage: Part A for hospitalization, Part B for services and supplies, Part C for filling the gaps between parts A and B, and Part D for prescription drugs. The costs associated for each part also vary on the basis of coverage and income levels. Part A is provided at no cost, and Part B can cost as little as nothing, but it increases in cost based on income levels. Parts C and D are administered by the private insurance market and vary given the coverage levels chosen. In essence, within our current Medicare system, Americans are given choice.

In Senator Sanders's plan, instead of choices, Americans will be offered "one-size-fits-all" coverage. This would encompass not only all health care and prescription drugs but also dental, vision, and long-term care. Sure, the thought of getting all of these things for "free" may sound good to the uninformed, but as most economists will tell you, everything costs something, and there's no such thing as "free." Senator Sanders has stated it's "a matter of principle," but to paraphrase James Carville, it's a matter of economy, stupid.

In 2017, the annual federal revenue paid to the US government was $3.3 trillion. While Senator Sanders claims his Medicare For All plan would cost between $1.2 trillion and $1.4 trillion, he hasn't actually produced any metrics as to how he's come up with that number. Several independent studies show the actual anticipated cost is closer to $3.26 trillion. Given those numbers, revenues would need to nearly double in order to pay for Medicare For All.

And when I say revenues, I mean *taxes*. Sure, the left can claim that they will tax only the rich, but let's be real: when it comes to new taxes, it's the middle class that suffers. The impact of Medicare For All would be extensive and would include the loss of jobs and the loss of innovation as well as the possible rationing of care.

Of the nearly 128 million employees in the United States, approximately 2.6 million are currently employed within the health care system; their jobs could be lost in a post-Medicare for All economy (1.5 million in health insurance, 1 million in hospital administration, and more than 81,000 in direct sales for pharmaceutical companies). Additionally, consider the call centers, technicians, facilities support, property management, real estate, custodial services, food services, and so forth, whose jobs are supported by the current health care structure.

And it's not just the jobs. The United States is responsible for the vast majority of medical innovation throughout the world. We advance medicine because of our free market ingenuity. If you want health care to *stop* advancing, then remove free market capitalism in the United States.

Regarding the rationing of care, I don't mean "death panels," but there would need to be a government entity that controls what claims and procedures would be approved or denied. Look no further than the United Kingdom to see that because of budget management, things like age, life expectancy, past life choices, and so forth impact who does and who doesn't get care.

These issues are all part of a single-payer system but not our current Medicare system. During his 2016 Presidential bid, Senator Sanders was a constant supporter of a "single payer" system that, according to Gallup, has only 31 percent favorability among Americans. Medicare users, however, report an 80 percent satisfaction rate, so, in effect, Democratic strategists have recognized that they have an issue of "name" versus "narrative." When you hear Democrats rally around Medicare For All, it's important to realize that this actually means single payer. Within the current proposals, there's very little Medicare at all.

The future of health care can hardly be called static in the best of times, and as we enter the next election cycle (during the writing of this book), health care is taking center stage once again. Democrats made significant political gains on health care during the 2018 midterms, taking back control of the House, and health care is quickly shaping up to be one of the primary deciding factors in the 2020 presidential election. According to Gallup, 80 percent of registered voters say that health care is extremely or very important to their vote, topping out as the number one issue for Democrats and the number three issue for Republicans.[89]

As discussed earlier, for many, there continue to be calls for a single-payer system or a public option. None of what has been proposed is viable, however, because of economics. Again, the current federal budget is $3.4 trillion, and the current single-payer options being floated have been estimated to cost approximately $3.2 trillion by several different organizations. The only way to shoehorn this single-payer system in would be either to reduce the current federal-spending level by 94 percent, leaving only 6 percent of the current budget, or to nearly double taxes to accommodate such a massive system. Both of these options are unfeasible and unlikely.

As we have outlined previously, many polls show possible support for a public option. Current polling by the KFF reveals the public likes the idea of a single-payer system, because the public appears to be slightly misinformed. This isn't a surprise; calling most of these plans a version of Medicare (which is a very popular program) evokes positive emotions by piggybacking off of the existing program. When Americans are asked if they would favor guaranteed health insurance as a right for them all, 71 percent approve of that right. But when Americans discover that guaranteed health insurance would threaten the current Medicare program and eliminate private health care, that approval number plummets to 32 percent. When Americans hear that single payer would also lead to delays in people receiving medical tests and treatment, that approval number plummets to 26 percent.[90] That's the power of good marketing: a forty-five point difference at the outset, until Americans find out what single payer really means.

So what could be some of the compromises? If not single payer, how about a public insurance option offered by the government, similar to that of other countries that have both public and private options, such as Germany? A variant of a Medicare and Medicaid buy-in shows strong approval among Americans when the eligibility age of Medicare is extended to a point between the ages of fifty and sixty-four. Republicans approve of such an extension by 69 percent, Independents, by 75 percent, and Democrats, by 85 percent,[91] averaging 77 percent approval. While I'm not advocating for a public option, compromise is possible; it's merely a matter of finding the middle ground.

The Middle Ground

A possible compromise that has been floated recently would be to expand the current Medicare system to include children—providing health care for all children under the age of 18. This certainly has some potential, because not only is it appealing to the public, it's actually financially feasible, unlike single payer. That's because health care for children is fairly straightforward. The average child's trips to the doctor are fairly routine, focused on things like preventative care, vaccines, physicals, colds and flu, setting broken bones, and so forth. This results in a far lower-cost average than adults, whose average medical costs increase annually the entirety of their lives.

Unlike the Medicare For All plans being touted by progressives, if we as a society are to offer up government-provided access to health insurance, we *must* be able to show how it can be paid for—anything less would be irresponsible. When it comes to expanding Medicare to include children, we've actually done the math and can show how it could be paid for in an easy-to-read way, with all of our sources published. Since this is for children, remember that, in school (but not always politics), you have to show your work!

Below you'll find a breakdown of the average cost by age and of the total population of those ages. By multiplying the total population by the average cost, we can get a rough estimate of what providing health care coverage to every child in the United States would cost. Here are the numbers:

- *Child Population of the United Sates—73,947,202*
- *Average Cost of Care per Year—$2,577.00*
- *Approximately six out of ten children of the US population of children are already enrolled in Medicaid or Medicare.*
    - *Currently Enrolled in Medicare/Medicaid—47,521,500*
    - *NOT currently enrolled—26,425,702*
- Multiplying the remaining 26,425,702 by $2,577.00 equals **$68,099,033,910.**

On the basis of the math provided above, **$68 billion** is the magic number in order to provide coverage to *all* children in the United States. But of course, this is America where when something becomes subsidized by the government (e.g., taxpayers), the cost of the item skyrockets. Additionally, we're relying on government reporting for our data. Let's say the government's numbers are all lowballed. If they are, we need to artificially inflate the numbers by, let's say, around a quarter more than we had expected. As my father would say, we should hope for the best but plan for the worst. That brings us to **$89,263,414,500**, which is no small number, but I'm a deficit hawk. I believe in balancing the scales. Thanks to our friends at the Congressional Budget Office (CBO), they provide nonpartisan data analysis to show how we could find the money for this project. All of the numbers I provide below are based on current ten-year averages. If we are to implement something as massive as this, we must find $89 billion to do so. These are just a few suggestions of where to find the money:

- **General Budget Reduction/Transfer**
  One of the easiest ways to provide for a project of such a scale is to look at the federal income as a whole. Utilizing a 1 percent reduction in overall spending and redirecting that number to providing health care for children would provide **$34 billion.** Even .5 percent reduction in spending would provide **$17 billion**.[92]

- **Defense Spending**
  It's too easy in the minds of some to go after the defense budget. The largest portion of our discretionary spending ($600 billion), it's a ripe target. That said, no one should want to weaken our defenses or "stick it" to our soldiers. With this in mind, here may be a reasonable request. This past year, the president boosted spending on defense by $61 billion, which the Department of Defense did not ask for. Since it's too easy to try to "take that back," we could ask for a modest 2 percent reduction in spending, or **12 billion**.[93]

- **Cannabis Taxation**
  While I recognize that legalizing marijuana is a touchy subject for many, given the idea of using revenues to help

children, such legalization might be a viable option. I'm not here to debate the morality of the issue; I'm here to try to find ways we can provide health care to children in need. That said, if we could do something good (and possibly hurt the drug cartel business, in the process), we should, at the very least, consider the option. According to the Pew Research Center, 62 percent of Americans favor marijuana legalization. On the basis of research from New Frontier Data, an analytics firm focused on the cannabis industry, if marijuana were to be legalized nationally and taxed at 15 percent, it would generate **$13.2 billion** per year, and around a half a million new jobs to boot[94] (and the jobs are just an added bonus).

- **Motor Fuel Indexing**
  Historically, gasoline prices are not being taxed to match inflation. This is an obviously popular move among politicians, as refusing to raise taxes on gasoline helps gets you reelected, but it does long-term damage to the system as a whole. If we were to increase excise taxes on motor fuels and index them for inflation, it would show that the United States is roughly thirty-five cents per gallon shy of what taxes on gasoline should be. Since I don't want to discourage travel and as someone who myself benefits from keeping prices low, perhaps we can meet less than halfway, and ask for a fifteen-cent tax on gasoline prices (it's for the children, right?). This adjustment still means that our tax rate on fuel is 58 percent less than what the CBO says it should be. Those fifteen cents would account for **$23.7 billion** in new revenue. Or if we went to full capacity and raised the tax to thirty-five cents per gallon (which I personally wouldn't like to see), that would generate **$51.4 billion**.[95]

- **Carbon Taxation**
  Carbon tax is a greenhouse gasses emissions tax. A good portion of First World countries have a tax for such emissions, and if we look at our cousins across the pond, we see that, in the European Union, that tax sits at $25USD per ton released into the atmosphere. Such a tax would raise over **$107 billion**, *but* it would be a massive strain on our economy and a huge shock to many of the companies that do business in the United States, not to mention that many of my Texas neighbors would uninvite me to their Christmas parties if I even suggested this. But remember that we're only trying to find money or ways to pay for health care coverage, so if a carbon tax is an option, perhaps we can meet at one-third of the EU tax, or $8.25 per emission ton. That's vastly less than our neighbors, but this still produces a large amount of revenue, **$35.97 billion**.[96]

- **Medicare Eligibility Adjustment**
  Another possibility is to raise the eligibility age of Medicare to sixty-seven. In 1965, when Medicare was created, the average life expectancy for an American was 70.25 years.[97] Medicare was intended to support people in their final few years, a noble purpose, as it is today.[98] That said, thanks to great advances in medical care and scientific research, the average life expectancy in 2019 is 78.8 years.[99] Instead of providing care for three to five years, Medicare is now providing care for thirteen to fifteen years. By raising the eligibility by two years, we would still double the number of years for which the program was initially intended. This two-year increase would provide, on average, **$5.5 billion** for the first ten years, and, after that, it would provide, on

average, **$15 to $20 billion** per year, throughout its usage by the baby boomer population.[100]

- **New Taxes**
  When all else fails, tax. I'm not trying to sound like George H. W. Bush and promise no new taxes, but perhaps increasing the current income tax rate for *all* Americans by 1 percent could be a fair trade-off in exchange for health care coverage for 100 percent of our child population. I mean, imagine how much removing this burden from American families would spur the economy (talk about your trickle-down economics). While I, by no means, like the idea of paying any more of my hard-earned money to the government, if we increased the current tax rate by 1 percent, we generate **$34 billion** in new revenue.

Summary

There you have it. While I'm not endorsing a "Medicare For All Children," it can be done and paid for. I've outlined seven options that, even in their limited state, could potentially raise a total amount of at least **$186 billion**, but if expanded to their recommended CBO modifications, they could allow for as much as **$260 billion**. Given that the program would cost approximately $89 billion to implement, these figures, at their minimum, allow for an excess of approximately $97 billion, which could be kept in their current place, be invested, or pooled for extraneous costs.

There are also intangible aspects to providing health care for children as well. Many of you reading this are parents, or will be someday. Imagine the relief of knowing your child will always have emergency care and that if you want to take that job leap or you want to make that move, that safety net would always be there for them. I know that when I formed my own company, providing for my family was, at the time, both the biggest motivator and the biggest terror in my life. Imagine how many entrepreneurs aren't creating new businesses, how many possible jobs are not coming to fruition because of the stranglehold that health care has on them. Lack of security is often cited as one of the principle reasons people are afraid to start a new business, and health care falls into that category.[101] It's one thing to be willing to go sick and hungry; it's another thing entirely to risk your children to suffer that fate as well.

In the end, there can be compromise when it comes to health care. Some may despise the idea of expanding our current government programs, and some may suggest that extending Medicare to children only does not go far enough. Either way, compromise can be accomplished and paid for—this is merely one suggestion.

CHAPTER 12

The Real Solution

Throughout this book, we have discussed many of the various problems within our current health care system. We have quantified the challenges created by those issues and have recommended a number of solutions that I believe could make a significant impact and begin moving us in the right direction. But there is one key component that absolutely must be involved at a much higher level than ever before if we want to cure health care: you.

An Analogy

I want you to take a moment and imagine you are entering a grocery store and grabbing a cart, maybe with a list of items needed for the week (if you're like me, that list was likely provided by your spouse). As you navigate the aisles, you maintain a confidence in the quality of the goods you are purchasing and a basic idea of what they will cost you. Once everything has been gathered, you make your way to the checkout aisle. The groceries begin to be scanned, and the price registers on the screen above. After all the goods have been bagged, you pay the balance due and walk out the door, receipt in hand and armed with the knowledge of the cost and the quality of the experience. Does this sound familiar?

Now, I want you to imagine that same grocery store, except that this time, as you make your way through the aisles, you begin to notice that there are no labels on any of the products. You also begin to notice that there are no prices listed, either. Needing groceries anyway, you continue to fill your basket, and just as you did before, you proceed to the checkout aisle, but, this time, as the products are scanned, you notice that there is no total showing up on the screen. Confused, you ask the clerk, "What is this going to cost me?" To your surprise, the clerk responds by asking which credit card company you intend to use to pay for the groceries. After telling the clerk, he or she then tells you that they will send the list of items you were purchasing to that specific credit card company and that you will receive a bill in roughly one to three months. Shaking your head, you take your groceries and walk out the door.

The first scenario I laid out seemed pretty common, right? It's not unlike an experience that we would have in any retail environment, whether it be groceries, clothing, electronics, or anything else, but this second scenario seems a bit crazy, doesn't it? We would never imagine going into a store to buy something without knowing what it would cost. But while it may seem far-fetched, if I would replace the grocery store with the US health care system, this scenario doesn't seem that unordinary.

The One with All The Power

Throughout this book, we've discussed the various parts of the health care system. We've outlined the players and the game they play in delivering, financing, and profiteering from the health care Americans consume. We've discussed the government's role in being the referee and setting the boundaries of how our free market economic system can not only continue to thrive but also can continue to be fair. The one key piece to all of this is the most important influencer of all and, in my opinion, the one with the most control—**YOU**.

In a free market system, the consumer is meant to have the power. In the United States, the consumer controls which restaurants remain open, which TV shows get renewed for a new season, which city professional sports teams reside in, even who becomes president of the United States. Yes, we, the consumers, have the power, yet when it comes to health care, we are too quick to yield that power and instead have found ourselves the pawns. But we can overcome—we can begin the movement to cure our health care system in the United States—we just have to pay attention and shift the way we think, approach, consume, and pay for health care. And here's how:

Let's revisit the economic principle we discussed early on. To restate the definition of "the economic principal": the true cost of something is equal to the number of units consumed multiplied by their price. Americans recognize this principle and apply it each and every day. If our electric bill is too high in winter, maybe we turn down the thermostat or shop for another provider. If our cable bill is too expensive, perhaps we turn off the sports package or premium channels. In times of increased fuel prices, Americans will do things like waiting in line for a lower cost, carpooling, or even ride a bike. The number of units consumed multiplied by their price is our cost—we apply this in all aspects of our consumer life, and the same should apply in our approach to health care, too.

We need to do our research ahead of time and not wait until we're in the heat of the moment. We should know which doctor should be our doctor, which hospital our hospital, and which drug does or doesn't have a generic or biosimilar—these decisions should be based on costs, quality, outcomes, and reviews. The information is out there—you just have to look—it's often accessible on the internet. Americans spend more than ten hours researching a car before they make their purchase and two hours researching a flat-screen TV, but when it comes to our health care, we spend, on average, only fifteen minutes.

Which brings me to my next point—*Ask questions.* In today's health care environment, a trip to our doctor seems more like a speed-dating round than one where we really want to understand or learn. Doctors are knowledgeable, but when it comes to your health, you should be, too. We don't gain knowledge or understanding by being quiet—we do so by speaking up. And when it comes to cost, questions could be your best friend—*Words are currency.* Our health care system doesn't operate on an outcomes basis; remember, it operates on a fee-for-service. The more tests you get, the more drugs you use, the more people you see, the more revenue is generated (regardless of the outcome). You should be on the front line, asking what each test, each drug, and each doctor is responsible for—you just might find you don't need quite as many units of health care as they may offer.

And, to that point, stop thinking about health care and health insurance as the same thing—they aren't. As I mentioned before, health insurance is just the financing mechanism of the health care delivery system, yet we've been trained to think about copays and deductibles as our cost, not the entirety of our purchase. News flash—health insurance companies aren't interested in taking a loss—whatever you cost them, they will get back. In life, there are things we finance—big-ticket items like homes and cars, but we'd never finance milk, eggs, and fabric softener. In the same way, we don't finance small stuff in health care, either—by running everything through our insurance. We'd never pay for an oil change with our auto insurance, so why are we paying for our cold and sinus medication with our health insurance? If we would begin thinking about health insurance premiums like amortization schedules on our mortgage, we might think differently about how we use our health insurance card. Health insurance isn't the solution; it's the credit card. Remember, there's a reason our ID cards look like a credit card.

And once you've received care, always ask for a line-item bill. If you will recall from an earlier chapter, studies have shown that 80 percent of medical bills contain errors (not typically in your favor). I couldn't imagine paying a bill that wasn't right, but so often, Americans do this every day. You'll be amazed at what you discover when viewing a medical bill. My favorite was the mucus recovery device listed at $8.00 per unit (by the way, that's a tissue). Health care billings are ridiculous, and this is mainly caused by two things.

1. Americans don't ask for a line-item bill.
2. We think about only what we have to pay before insurance.

Remember: today's insurance claims become tomorrow's premiums, so make sure the entire bill is right. In the end, you're paying it, anyway.

And, finally, be confident—you are smarter than the insurance companies give you credit for, but when it comes to health care, unfortunately, we're often as lazy as they make us out to be. Remember this: doctors, hospitals, pharmaceutical companies, insurers—they are working for you—they are vying for your business; you are their customer. *So act like it.*

Health care is a problem in the United States, no doubt, and fixing it seems like a daunting task. All those involved will need to play their parts, but it all begins and ends with you. You are the solution. Remember the economic principle, do your research, ask the questions, think about what you are financing, review your costs, and be confident.

Our health care system in the United States is amazing on the whole; doctors, hospitals, and those working within them are good people and want to do good things. The people working at the pharmaceutical companies want to develop new drugs to improve the quality and the longevity of life. People are inherently good. I believe that, but health care is also a business, no different than the ice cream shop, the grocery store, the clothing store, or the cable company. Those in business want to make money, and they should. With that money, they provide jobs and the services we want and need. If those businesses weren't profitable, they wouldn't be around and available to all of us. But in our free market system, we, the consumers, are ultimately the regulating power. Sure, we need Uncle Sam to set and govern the rules, but always remember that health care, in all of its greatness, is a business—approach it that way. Be diligent, be confident, be a consumer, and together, *we* will be the cure to health care.

Notes

1 ps://khn.org/news/15-minute-doctor-visits/
2 https://www.cms.gov/Outreach-and-Education/Medicare-Learning-Network-MLN/MLNProducts/downloads/medcrephysfeeschedfctsht.pdf
3 https://www.nhpf.org/library/the-basics/Basics_RVUs_01-12-15.pdf (Used to demonstrate updating of RVU Values)
4 https://books.google.com/books?hl=en&lr=&id=tD6Y5oUIQAoC&oi=fnd&pg=PR1&ots=ZfU3-7xDLt&sig=E9_6Z94pn2AHNa_ZiATPh54-1Tw#v=onepage&q&f=false (Medical Decision Making)
5 https://conciergemedicinenews.files.wordpress.com/2016/03/infog-dpc-4-3.jpg (Concierge Better Relationship)
6 https://news.aamc.org/medical-education/article/new-aamc-research-reaffirms-looming-physician-shor/ (Shortage of PCP Estimates)
7 https://www.ncbi.nlm.nih.gov/pmc/articles/PMC2150598/ (Multiple Comorbidities in Elderly)
8 https://www.nytimes.com/2016/10/25/upshot/why-the-us-still-trails-many-wealthy-nations-in-access-to-care.html?module=inline (Extra Doctors Needed Due to ACA)
9 https://news.gallup.com/poll/195086/uninsured-down-obamacare-cost-quality-concerns.aspx?g_source=uninsured&g_medium=search&g_campaign=tiles (Using ACA metrics)
10 https://www.healthcostinstitute.org/research/annual-reports (Healthcare Utilization Metrics)

11 https://www.studentdebtrelief.us/news/average-medical-school-debt/ (Averages of Medical School Debt)
12 https://www.ahrq.gov/research/findings/factsheets/primary/pcwork1/index.html (Breakdown of Practicing PCPs in the US)
13 https://www.cdc.gov/nchs/injury/index.htm (CDC Tracking of Visits)
14 http://www.annfammed.org/content/7/2/104.full (Type of injury for doctor Usage)
15 https://slate.com/business/2018/08/nyu-medical-school-plans-free-tuition-for-all-what-a-waste-of-money.html (What a Waste Quote)
16 https://www.insidehighered.com/admissions/article/2019/01/14/nyu-medical-school-sees-surge-applications-after-going-tuition-free (Increases in NYU diversity after free tuition.)
17 https://www.ncbi.nlm.nih.gov/pmc/articles/PMC4229497/ (Medical Student Debt and Major Life Choices Survey)
18 https://www.medscape.com/features/slideshow/public/residents-salary-and-debt-report-2015 (Residency Average Income)
19 https://www.nejm.org/doi/full/10.1056/NEJMp0903460#t=article (Average Incomes of Specialists)
20 https://www.nejm.org/doi/full/10.1056/NEJMp0903460#t=article (6 Million Extra over Course of Career)
21 https://fas.org/sgp/crs/misc/R44970.pdf (NHSC Statistics)
22 https://www.beckershospitalreview.com/workforce/nursing-schools-reject-thousands-of-applicants-amid-shortage.html (Comment on lack of funding for applicants spots)
23 https://revcycleintelligence.com/news/less-than-a-third-of-docs-owned-independent-practices-in-2018
24 http://www.physiciansadvocacyinstitute.org/Portals/0/assets/docs/2016-PAI-Physician-Employment-Study-Final.pdf
25 https://www.advisory.com/daily-briefing/2018/11/15/hospital-mergers

26 https://www.strategyand.pwc.com/media/file/Size-should-matter.pdf

27 https://www.healthaffairs.org/doi/pdf/10.1377/hlthaff.22.6.88

28 https://www.advisory.com/daily-briefing/2018/11/15/hospital-mergers

29 http://petris.org/resources/ (Link to the publications available)

30 https://www.ncci.com/Articles/Pages/II_Insights_QEB_Impact-of-Hospital-Consolidation-on-Medical-Costs.aspx

31 Dafny, Leemore, "Estimation and Identification of Merger Effects: An Application to Hospital Mergers," 5 52.3 (2009): 523-550.

32 Capps, Cory and David Dranove, "Hospital Consolidation and Negotiated PPO Prices," *Health Affairs*23.2 (2004): 175-181.

33 https://www.justice.gov/atr/case/us-v-mercy-health-services-and-finley-tri-states-health-group-inc

34 https://law.justia.com/cases/federal/district-courts/FSupp/707/840/1574626/

35 https://www.mercatus.org/conlaws (lists the rules attendant to each of the 35 states with CON laws)

36 https://www.modernhealthcare.com/article/20181203/NEWS/181209987/white-house-urges-states-to-repeal-certificate-of-need-laws (Trump administration supporting repeal of CON laws.)

37 https://www.hhs.gov/sites/default/files/Reforming-Americas-Healthcare-System-Through-Choice-and-Competition.pdf

38 https://en.wikipedia.org/wiki/Hanlon%27s_razor

39 http://www.healthcarebusinesstech.com/medical-billing/ (4/5 Bills contain errors)

40 https://www.employeebenefitadviser.com/opinion/why-clients-should-care-about-medical-billing-errors-and-what-they-should-do-about-it?regconf=1 (Equifax Billing Errors)

41 https://www.forbes.com/sites/kateashford/2014/08/15/challenging-a-medical-bill/#105eae482342 (Victoria Caras Quote)

42 https://khn.org/news/the-remedy-for-surprise-medical-bills-may-lie-in-stitching-up-federal-law/ (18% Statistic)

43 https://www.commonwealthfund.org/sites/default/files/documents/___media_files_publications_issue_brief_2017_jun_lucia_balance_billing_ib.pdf (ER to blame for Balance Billing)

44 https://www.beckershospitalreview.com/finance/20-things-to-know-about-balance-billing.html (70% oon statistic)

45 https://www.dallasnews.com/business/health-care/2018/08/28/after-heart-attack-texas-teacher-now-faces-108951-balance-bill-twice-annual-pay (Drew Calver Quote)

46 https://capitol.texas.gov/BillLookup/History.aspx?LegSess=86R&Bill=SB1264 (Texas Legislation Balance Bills)

47 https://www.tdi.texas.gov/consumer/cpmmediation.html (Balance Billing TDI)

48 http://bettertexasblog.org/author/spogue/ (Stacey Pogue Quote)

49 https://www.fool.com/retirement/2017/05/01/this-is-the-no-1-reason-americans-file-for-bankrup.aspx (Cause of bankruptcy Medical Debt)

50 https://ajph.aphapublications.org/doi/10.2105/AJPH.2018.304901?eType=EmailBlastContent&eId=a5697b7e-8ffc-4373-b9d2-3eb745d9debb&=& (AJPH Quote)

51 https://www.kff.org/report-section/the-burden-of-medical-debt-section-3-consequences-of-medical-bill-problems/ (Quotes on Medical Debt)

52 https://www.google.com/finance/UNH (United Healthcare Stock)

53 https://www.google.com/finance/ANTM (BCBS Stock)

54 https://www.google.com/search?q=CIGNA+stock&oq=CIGNA+STOCK&aqs=chrome.0.69i59j0l5.1240j1j9&sourceid=chrome&ie=UTF-8 (CIGNA Stock)

55 https://www.marketplace.org/2009/07/23/business/fallout-financial-crisis/cleveland-clinic-model-success (Pres. Obama quote)

56 https://www.thehealthlawfirm.com/resources/health-law-articles-and-documents/Beware-legal-ramifications-of-unnecessary-tests.html

57 https://www.justice.gov/opa/pr/missouri-hospital-system-agrees-pay-93-million-resolve-false-claims-act-and-stark-law

58 https://www.thehealthlawfirm.com/blog/posts/doctors-under-pressure-to-meet-quotas-and-fill-hospital-beds.html

59 https://revcycleintelligence.com/news/understanding-the-basics-of-bundled-payments-in-healthcare

60 https://my.clevelandclinic.org/health/articles/15938-value-based-care (Value-Based Care Cleveland Clinic)

61 https://ftp.cdc.gov/pub/Health_Statistics/NCHS/NHIS/SHS/2017_SHS_Table_A-18.pdf (Adults Visiting Doctors Stats)

62 https://ftp.cdc.gov/pub/Health_Statistics/NCHS/NHIS/SHS/2017_SHS_Table_C-8.pdf (Children Visiting Doctors Stats)

63 https://www.statista.com/statistics/238702/us-total-medical-prescriptions-issued/ (Total Rx Issued)

64 https://www.actuary.org/content/prescription-drug-spending-us-health-care-system (Total Rx Spent $)

65 https://www.snopes.com/fact-check/cocaine-coca-cola/ (Coca-Cola Cocaine)

66 https://www.fda.gov/about-fda/fda-basics/when-and-why-was-fda-formed (FDA Creation)

67 https://arstechnica.com/science/2019/01/healthcare-industry-spends-30b-on-marketing-most-of-it-goes-to-doctors/ (29.9b spent on Medical Advertising.)

68 https://www.bbc.com/news/business-28212223 (Johnson & Johnson R&D / Profit Statements)

69 https://www.sciencedirect.com/science/article/abs/pii/S0167629616000291#! (2.6 Billion Dollars New Drugs)

70 https://www.fda.gov/regulatory-information/search-fda-guidance-documents/acceptance-foreign-clinical-studies (FDA World Medical Association Declaration Changes)

71 https://www.wma.net/who-we-are/leaders/ (World Medical Association Leaders)

72 https://www.fda.gov/patients/drug-development-process/step-3-clinical-research (FDA Clinical Trial Length)

73 https://www.pcrsnetwork.com/2015/10/30/the-value-of-getting-a-new-drug-to-market-quicker/ (712k per day)

74 https://www.forbes.com/sites/tomasphilipson/2014/02/03/dont-be-fooled-brand-drugs-cut-prices-more-than-generics/#37fc0bc2113f (Generic and Market Share Devaluation)

75 https://www.forbes.com/sites/brucejapsen/2016/07/21/how-abbvies-humira-undercuts-the-drug-industry-price-defense/#232237206821 (Humira Annual Cost)

76 http://www.ncpa.co/pdf/PBM-Storybook-6pg.pdf (What Is a PBM)

77 https://www.statista.com/statistics/215479/price-change-of-leading-brand-drugs-in-the-us/ (1010 Percent Increase Stat)

78 https://jamanetwork.com/journals/jama/article-abstract/2545691#jsc160015r8 (Medicare Buying Power)

79 https://www.investopedia.com/investing/which-industry-spends-most-lobbying-antm-so/ (Lobby Size)

80 https://www.congress.gov/bill/108th-congress/house-bill/1 (MMA 2003)

81 https://www.nytimes.com/2010/02/13/health/policy/13pharm.html (Billy Tauzin Salary)

82 https://www.opensecrets.org/members-of-congress/industries?cid=N00000781&cycle=CAREER (Frank Pallone Campaign Donations)

83 https://fred.stlouisfed.org/series/MEPAINUSA672N (Average Income US Census)

84 https://en.wikipedia.org/wiki/United_States_House_Committee_on_Energy_and_Commerce (Total Members)

85 https://www.opensecrets.org/lobby/indusclient.php?id=H04&year=2019 (Health Industry Lobbying)

86 https://www.kff.org/health-costs/poll-finding/kaiser-health-tracking-poll-august-2015/ (KFF Poll Lobbying)

87 http://www.cbo.gov/sites/default/files/cbofiles/attachments/49638-BudgetOptions.pdf#page=59 (CBO Savings on Part D Negotiations)

88 https://www.crfb.org/press-releases/fact-sheet-how-much-money-could-medicare-save-negotiating-prescription-drug-prices (Secretary Ability to Negotiate Statement)

89 https://news.gallup.com/poll/244367/top-issues-voters-healthcare-economy-immigration.aspx (Gallup Poll)

90 https://www.kff.org/slideshow/public-opinion-on-single-payer-national-health-plans-and-expanding-access-to-medicare-coverage/ Medicare for All Poll

91 https://www.kff.org/health-reform/poll-finding/kff-health-tracking-poll-january-2019/ (Medicare Buy-In Poll)

92 https://www.nationalpriorities.org/budget-basics/federal-budget-101/spending/ (Federal Budget)

93 https://www.thebalance.com/u-s-military-budget-components-challenges-growth-3306320 (Defense Spending)

94 https://newfrontierdata.com/product/us-economy-2018/ Cannabis Taxes

95 https://www.cbo.gov/budget-options/2018/54817 (Motor Fuel Indexing)

96 https://www.cbo.gov/budget-options/2018/54821 (Carbon Tax)

97 http://www.demog.berkeley.edu/~andrew/1918/figure2.html (Average Life Expectancy 1965)

98 https://www.ourdocuments.gov/doc.php?flash=true&doc=99 (Purpose of Medicare)

99 https://gerontology.usc.edu/resources/infographics/americans-are-living-longer/ (Life Expectancy 2019)

100 https://www.cbo.gov/budget-options/2018/54733)Medicare to 67

101 https://medium.com/swlh/if-you-want-to-be-an-entrepreneur-dont-expect-to-have-these-5-things-in-your-life-4eb93da15381 (Entrepreneur Stability)